SEXUAL
HEALING
THROUGH
YIN &
YANG

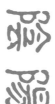

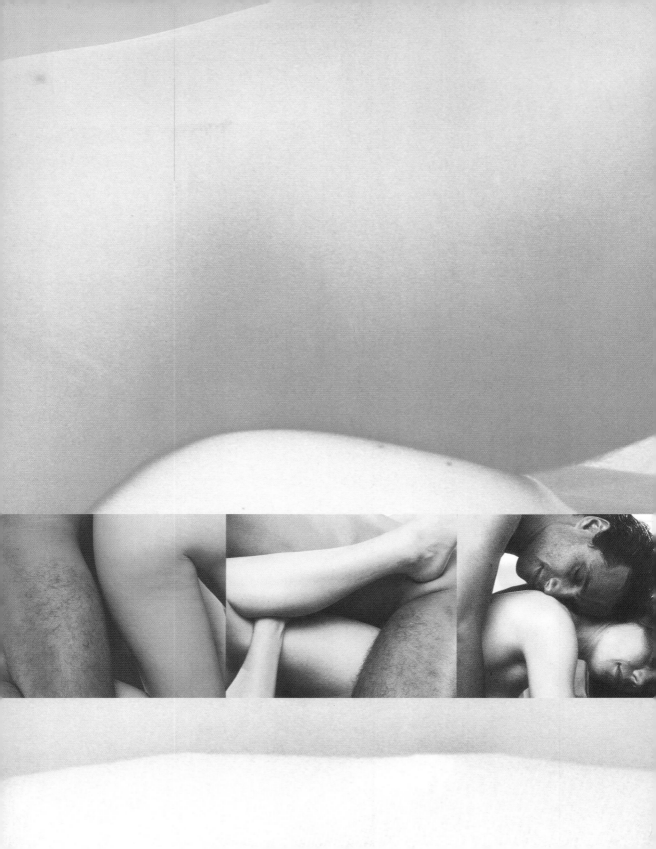

SEXUAL HEALING THROUGH YIN & YANG

ZAIHONG SHEN

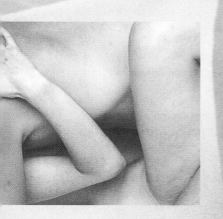
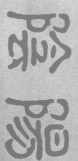
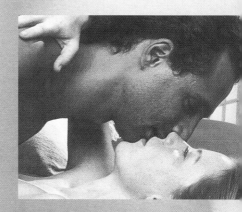

A DORLING KINDERSLEY BOOK

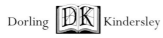

Dorling **DK** Kindersley

LONDON, NEW YORK, SYDNEY, DEHLI, PARIS,
MUNICH, and JOHANNESBURG

Project Editors: LaVonne Carlson and Barbara M. Berger
Developmental Editor: Stephanie Pedersen
Book Designer: Claire Legemah
Cover Art Director: Dirk Kaufman
Photographer: Kellie Walsh
Indexer: Nanette Cardon

Category Publisher: LaVonne Carlson
Art Director: Tina Vaughan
Senior Art Editor: Mandy Earey
Assistant Editor: Crystal A. Coble
DTP Designer: Jill Bunyan
Picture Researcher: Jo Walton
Production: Elizabeth Cherry, Joanna Bull
Assistant Picture Editor: Laarnie Ragaza

First American Edition, 2001
00 01 02 03 04 05 10 9 8 7 6 5 4 3 2 1
Published in the United States by
Dorling Kindersley Publishing, Inc.
95 Madison Avenue
New York, New York 10016

DK Publishing offers special discounts for bulk purchases for sales
promotions or premiums. Specific, large-quantity needs can be met
with special editions, including personalized covers, excerpts of
existing guides, and corporate imprints. For more information, contact
Special Markets Department, DK Publishing, Inc., 95 Madison Avenue,
New York, NY 10016
Fax: 800-600-9098.

A Cataloging in Publication record is available upon request
ISBN 0-7894-6769-0

Color reproduction by Colourscan, Singapore
Printed and bound in Hong Kong

See our complete catalog at
www.dk.com

CONTENTS

PART ONE
ROOTS OF SEXUAL HEALING THROUGH YIN & YANG 10

PART TWO
SEXUAL YIN & YANG: THE BASICS 28

FOREWORD

EALING Through Yin and Yang is a refreshingly different look at sex and sexual health, examined through the medium of the historic, scientific, and spiritual character of an ancient people. The more we learn about the ancients, from gene research and from reconstruction of their way of life, the more we discover that there was little if any difference between their intelligence and physical ability and ours. The main thing that has altered between then and now is technology.

I write about these facts for the scoffers—those who believe that there is nothing to be learned from men and women who crumbled into dust eons ago. The scoffers are wrong. A new perspective (new for us, that is) is always valuable. I've been fascinated to learn from these pages, for example, that the ancient Chinese believed severe weather conditions adversely affect the experience of sex. Bearing in mind severe weather is likely to be caused by fluctuation in the Earth's magnetic and electrical fields, this could make a lot of sense. And yet it's not something we Westerners would normally give the time of day. Perhaps we should. If you are an enthusiast of Feng Shui you will already believe that certain Earth fluctuations influence our senses. This book is a kind of Feng Shui of sex!

I loved the idea, expounded in these pages, that sex can be used to heal certain physical conditions. The penis and vagina (particularly the vagina) are believed to contain certain meridian points, which if stimulated, provoke change in specific sites elsewhere on the body. Readers are probably already aware that acupuncture works by moving energy from one part of the body to another in order to rebalance it through stimulating meridian points on more traditional body sites. According to Taoist belief sexual intercourse does the same, since it presses on the genital meridians.

In my own book *The Ultimate Sex Guide* I referred to the Taoist idea of The Sets of Nine where a certain type of prolonged intercourse was supposed to stimulate just about every sexual meridian you might think of, resulting in a thoroughly well balanced body with energy humming along in every limb, just as it should. If you think about it, most of you will confess to feeling exceedingly well at the end of a successful love-making, as if the whole body has been worked out. The only place where I differ from the Taoists is that I think orgasm is a necessary part of the rebalancing process. Which is not to say that the ancient Chinese believed you should never climax. But they found a lot of reasons why it might be a good idea to climax less frequently.

The explanation usually given for this is the belief that orgasm will dissipate energy, as indeed it does, but to my mind with pleasurable results. But it occurs to me that the ancient Chinese didn't have too much in the way of reliable contraception. It might have been in everyone's interest that men conserved their orgasmic emission as much as possible so, by formulating such a positive healing by-product of so doing (ie. good sexual health), a brilliant teaching method was born.

Yet we would do well to read the healing sections of Healing Through Yin and Yang with care. It may sound faintly comic to have certain types of prolonged intercourse in order to cure, say, the flu, but suppose it actually works? Wouldn't this be a great way of taking medicine? I, for one, would love a remedy for athletic joint injuries and have decided to experiment with the Qiang Gu (exercise to strengthen the bones). Let's hope you'll see me out jogging again before long.

I was also glad to see references to the Chinese use of dildos. A dildo is the forerunner to the vibrator. In this book it is used for training and strengthening the vaginal muscles. In sex therapy today we actually use dildos to help women with vaginismus (a condition where the vagina goes into rigid spasm on intercourse), get used to the idea of penetration, and so to relax their attitude towards it. With the discovery and harnessing of electricity, 20th century humans have taken the dildo a step further. In this shape of the vibrator it can not only be used for all the ancient Chinese methods of sex therapy but can also be activated on the outside of the vagina and in particular on the clitoris. I don't have a single doubt that the Chinese with their incredible wisdom and profound sense of culture would have been the first to seize upon the erotic potential of electricity. So a small addition of my own to this excellent book is to suggest including the vibrator when you come to rebalancing your personal yin and yang.

I must confess to a flicker of doubt when I first read about the Iron Jade Stalk exercise, which involves repeatedly plunging the penis into a bowl of sand. But then, I reflected, even Buddhist monks are entitled to their little jokes! This is a truly thought-provoking book.

Anne Hooper

ABOUT SEXUAL HEALING THROUGH YIN & YANG

Sex—it's a biological necessity, needed to ensure the continuation of humankind. Yet in present-day America, sex is considered as recreational as it is procreational. In fact, sex could be seen as a national pastime: We read about it in the latest bestsellers, we watch it at the movie theater, we find advice for it in national magazines, we listen to other people's sexual tales on daytime television. Obviously, sex is a hot topic.

THE people of ancient China were as interested in sex as we are today. Emperors, empresses, princes, princesses, courtesans, healers, religious leaders, and philosophers debated the theories and practices of sensual pleasure, which lead to the creation of a number of now-classic sexual letters, memoirs, how-to manuals, songs, and poems. This detailed literature outlines everything from how to choose a lover to preparing an enticing environment, from gauging a partner's arousal to methods of extending orgasm. *Sexual Healing through Yin & Yang* includes much of

this information within 'Ancient Sex Basics' (page 58). Because strength, flexibility, and endurance were seen to enhance sensual pleasure, breathing and strengthening exercises were also regularly performed by both men and women. Look for these in 'Before Getting Started' (page 46).

Among the elite classes of ancient China, however, sex provided more than pleasure. Intercourse was used as a powerful healing tool. According to ancient Chinese theories, sex's healing power comes from yin energy and yang energy. In simplest terms, yin represents receptive (or feminine) energy, while yang represents generative (or masculine) energy. Every human body, regardless of gender, contains both yin and yang energy. Yin and yang energy coexist as equals within the body, though there are times when the delicate balance between the two types of energy is thrown off. Too much work, too much food, even too much intercourse are among the things that can upset the equilibrium of yin and yang. When this balance is upset, mental or physical illnesses, ranging from mild headaches to infertility to heart problems, are believed to occur.

Sexual Healing through Yin & Yang presents conditions that may occur when yin and yang are improperly balanced. The book offers ancient sexual prescriptions to restore equilibrium between yin and yang, thus returning the body to its balanced state. Known as 'Healing by the Lover' (page 130), these healing prescriptions go beyond a simple sexual position; Western readers will be surprised that many suggest a specific number of thrusts, wiggles, rotations, or other movements. Orgasm is not the goal of these positions; after performing the requisite number of moves, the exercise is over and the couple is advised to stop. Furthermore, the exercise may need to be repeated several times a day—each time with only the advised number of movements.

Those who believe 'prevention is the best medicine' will be happy to know that the old saying was as apt in ancient China as it is in latter-day America. It was the ancient Chinese belief in illness-prevention that prompted strict rules regarding the use of sex to ward off sickness. Found in 'Situations to Avoid' (page 34), these dictums include specific erotic positions that thwart given maladies, as well as an exacting list of times and conditions in which intercourse should be avoided altogether.

Finally, because conception is often the desired result of sex, the same exacting requirements are applied to reproduction. Therefore, anyone hoping to combine recreation, good health, and conception should turn to 'Reproductive Health' (page 44), which shares ancient information on improving fertility and safeguarding pregnancy.

Sexual Healing through Yin & Yang was designed as a reference guide for health-conscious individuals. If you believe you are ill, common sense dictates that you avoid self-diagnosis. Instead, contact a trusted healthcare provider to discuss any possible health problems. Applied responsibly, the information in *Sexual Healing through Yin & Yang* promises to show you another way of seeing and using sex: as an enjoyable, fun-spirited tool to help foster well-being. Use it in pleasure and health!

CHINESE ANATOMICAL TERMS

In Chinese literature, sexual positions and body parts are often referred to by poetic-sounding plant or animal names. Though we offer English terms throughout the book, the following are typical of terms used in Chinese literature:

Female genitalia Butterfly, Lily Flower

Woman on top Candle Light

Vagina Cinnabar Grotto, Dark River, Jade Gate

Upper vulva Golden Gulch

Lower vulva Jade Vein

Labia majora Jade Lips, Instrument String

Labia minora Coxcombs, Scarlet Pearls

Clitoris Animal in the Boat, Jewel Terrace, Red Pearl

Cervix Flower Pistil, Flower Heart

Uterus Scarlet Chamber

Penis Jade Stem, Jade Stalk

Testicles Eggs

Semen; Male and female sexual lubrication Jade Liquid

Man inserts his penis an inch into the vagina then withdraws Dragonfly, Lute Strings, Shallow Method

Man inserts his penis two inches into the vagina then withdraws Wheatbud

Man inserts his penis three inches into the vagina then withdraws Scented Mouse

Man inserts his penis four inches into the vagina then withdraws Mixed Rock

Man inserts his penis five inches into the vagina then withdraws Grain Seed

陰 陽

ROOTS
OF
SEXUAL
HEALING
THROUGH
YIN &
YANG

CHAPTER ONE

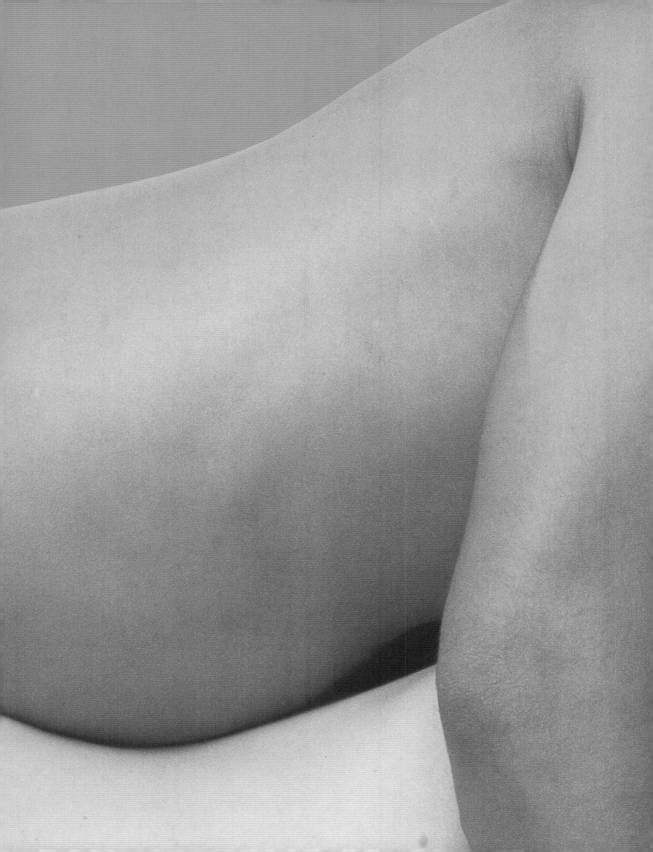

THE YIN & YANG METHOD

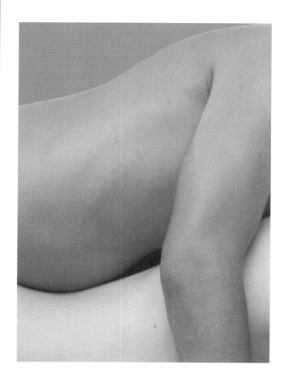

THE ANCIENT CHINESE BELIEVED
THAT GOOD SEX REQUIRED
PERFECT EQUILIBRIUM
BETWEEN YIN AND YANG.

HISTORY OF THE YIN & YANG METHOD

THE yin and yang method—the Chinese term for health-supportive sex—has been used in China even before the appearance of written language. The concept first appeared in print late in the Zhou dynasty (c. 1027-256 B.C.), when philosophers refined the concept of yin and yang and created the related theory of duality, encompassing heaven and earth, sun and moon, man and woman. According to yin and yang philosophy, since heaven turns left and the earth turns right, the man should be on top or to the left during sex and the woman should be underneath or to the right during sex.

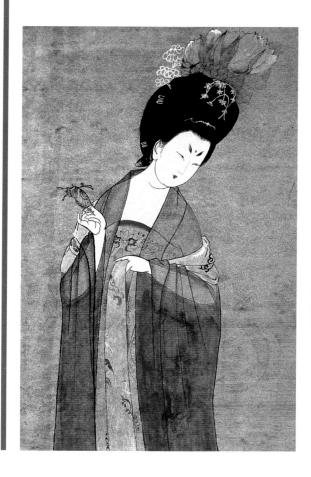

Since that time, the yin and yang method has been enthusiastically practiced in various dynasties—though not always with a ruler's consent. During the repressive Qin dynasty (221-207 B.C.), many earlier sexology texts were destroyed. But the health- and pleasure-seeking elite of ancient China did not forgo the 'art of the bedchamber'— another term for the yin and yang method. Instead, Chinese aristocrats quietly sought hidden sources of sexual information.

Some of the earliest publicly circulated stories concerning the yin and yang method originated during the Han dynasty (c. 207 B.C.-A.D. 220). The Han dynasty—sometimes divided into the earlier West Han and later East Han dynasties—is considered China's first long empirical dynasty, during which the country became widely known as 'China.' During this era, much previously banned literature was recorded and recopied. Anecdotes from the time include the emperor who ordered that an immense dish be built atop a 270-foot tower to collect dew, which he drank daily to increase his sexual stamina. It was also during this time that 'elixirs of immortality' became popular. Concocted by alchemists, these mixtures were consumed by Chinese royalty, government officials, aristocrats, scholars, and physicians to increase sexual prowess; the potions often contained any number of herbs, the dried and ground genitals of animals, pulverized birds nests, ground pearls, and cinnabar (a naturally occurring mercury sulfide).

CHINESE DYNASTY CHART

DYNASTY	TIME
Hsia	c. 1994-1523 B.C.
Shang	c. 1523-1027 B.C.
Zhou	1027-256 B.C.
Western Zhou	1027-770 B.C.
Eastern Zhou	770-256 B.C.
Qin	221-207 B.C.
Han	207 B.C.-A.D. 220
West Han	207 B.C.-A.D. 25
East Han	25-220 A.D.
Three Kingdoms	A.D. 220-265
Western Jin	A.D. 265-420
Six Dynasties	A.D. 420-589
Sui	A.D. 589-618
Tang	A.D. 618-906
Five Dynasties	A.D. 907-960
Song	A.D. 960-1279
Jin	A.D. 1115-1234
Yuan	A.D. 1279-1368
Ming	A.D. 1368-1644
Qing	A.D. 1644-1912

While some mixtures produced successful results, a number of blends containing cinnabar caused illness—or death—from mercury poisoning.

During the Tang dynasty (A.D. 618-907, known as China's 'Golden Age,' the art of the bedchamber flourished most openly. Taoism, with its belief in the health-giving properties of sex (that gave birth to the yin and yang method), was made the national religion. Further increasing the yin and yang method's popularity among the common people were the widely reported exploits of romantic Tang dynasty emperors. Hsuan Tsung (A.D. 718-761), for example, gathered potential partners together and placed a flower in each woman's hair.

THE FIRST HUMANS

One day the spirit-god Nu Wa was bored, so she fashioned some figures out of clay, modeling them after herself. When she blew her chi into them, they became living women (yin) and men (yang). Soon thereafter, the women and men began to reproduce by themselves. This is the Chinese myth of the first earthly reproduction through yin and yang.

He then released a butterfly. The woman whose flower attracted the butterfly would be the ruler's bedmate. Ching Tsung (A.D. 806-820) threw sachets of scented powder; whoever was hit by the perfume was his lady for the night. Cheng Tsung (A.D. 825-826) etched the first two lines of a popular four-line poem on a leaf and set the leaf adrift in the royal canal. Women were asked to inscribe the last two lines of a well-known poem on a leaf, which were set afloat in the same canal. When one of the women's leaves drifted alongside the emperor's, the two leaves were retrieved. If the emperor's first two lines and the lady's last two lines were from the same poem, the two spent the night together.

The freewheeling sex of the Tang dynasty was restrained during the Sung dynasty (A.D. 960-1279). The change in sexual climate is attributed to the rise of Confucianism, which advocated the inferiority of women, the segregation of the sexes, and the restriction of sex to procreation. Sexual poems were banned, visual works of erotic art and books of sexual literature were destroyed, and women were not allowed to speak to male non-relations unless hidden behind a screen. The masses and the women of China's elite classes were most affected; in the royal courts, male rulers continued having intercourse with thousands of women.

This 'prudishness' continued in the Ming dynasty (A.D. 1368-1644) and through the Qing or Manchu dynasty (A.D. 1644-1912). So serious were the Manchurians about sexual health that royal bed-

THE YELLOW EMPEROR

One of the most frequently recurring names in ancient Chinese sexology is Huang Ti, The Yellow Emperor, who ascended to the throne in 2697 B.C., during the legendary Age of the Five Rulers. The Yellow Emperor was so interested in strengthening and maintaining his health—reportedly to please the estimated 1200 women he slept with during his lifetime—that he commissioned a team of six doctors to work with him on a book of medicine. Called *Yellow Emperor's Inner Jing*, or *The Yellow Emperor's Classic of Internal Medicine*, the work is considered the first book of Chinese medicine. In it are theories of yin and yang, the five elements, chi and chi meridians, and acupressure and acupuncture.

According to Chinese legends, Huang Ti's great vitality and his contribution to Chinese medicine made him immortal. Instead of dying a mortal death, he was said to have ascended into heaven in daylight.

AN EXCERPT FROM THE CLASSIC OF THE ELEMENTAL LADY

In the opening passage of *The Classic of the Elemental Lady*, the Yellow Emperor is depressed and experiencing impotence. He asks Lady Su what he can do to feel better. She replies:

'The debility of men is caused by faulty ways in the mating of yin and yang. Women prevail over men, just as water prevails over fire. They that know the way are like a good cook who can blend the five flavors into a tasty soup. They that know the Tao of yin and yang can blend the five pleasures. But they that know not may die an untimely death. How could they ever enjoy sexual pleasures?.'

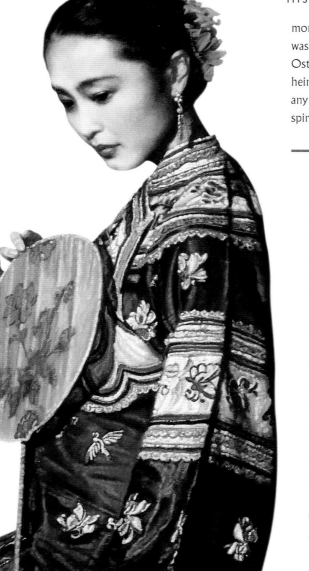

monitoring reached new heights: A royal eunuch was assigned to observe all royal sexual encounters. Ostensibly, this was to validate the authenticity of all heirs, but the eunuch could also stop the emperor at any time during sex if he deemed it too lengthy or spirited for the monarch's health.

THE FIRST SEXOLOGISTS

Ancient Chinese followers of Taoism believed that general health, well-being, and youth could be attained through a rich, fulfilling sex life. Among the earliest-known Taoist proponents of sex-for-health were three women: Su Nu, also known as the Elemental Lady; Hsuan Nu, or the Arcane Lady; and Tsai Nu, otherwise known as the Iridescent Lady.

Su Nu, the first and most widely quoted of the 'three ladies,' wrote a book during the first century A.D. that became known as *The Book of Lady Su* or *The Classic of the Elemental Lady*. In this book, Su Nu holds a discussion with the Yellow Emperor (who was actually deceased by this time) on using sex to strengthen the body's balance of yin and yang energy.

The works by Hsuan Nu and Tsai Nu, which were written shortly after Su Nu's text, were destroyed during China's Confucian period. Like Su Nu's book, Hsaun Nu's and Tsai Nu's stories were penned as conversations with the Yellow Emperor, a ruler interested in the link between sex and health. In addition to specific formulas to cure or prevent illnesses, these texts provided information on creating a sensual environment, foreplay, sustaining pleasure, and bringing a sexual partner to orgasm.

WORDS OF LOVE

POETRY—both reading and writing—was an important pastime in ancient China. While poetic verse was used to celebrate everything from holidays to religion, romantic poetry was especially popular. The following selections are typical of ancient Chinese love poems, particularly in their use of erotic allusion. Note that poems, including these, were not given titles.

THIS poem, taken from the *Jin Ping Mei*, depicts a sexual encounter between a man and a woman. Among the veiled sexual references in this poem are 'dark river,' which refers to the vagina; 'Butterfly' which was a euphemism for the entire female genitalia; and 'Dragonfly,' a sexual position in which a man used only very shallow thrusts during intercourse.

Silence, chamber, cold pillow,
The man and the beauty in wonderful heaven;
Red candles dripping the wax down,
All of a sudden the boat took a turn in
the dark river;
Butterfly steeling among the flowers,
Dragonfly playing the water up and down;
Ultimate happiness and intense
motion have no end,
The holy turtle spilt the spring water.

TAKEN from the *Jin Ping Mei*, this poem celebrates a garden where lovers once met.

Cherry Tree, deep garden, rain just stops,
Moss path, no wind, butterfly is free;

The hundred lilacs do not show
off their beauty,
Three strings of willow play softly;

Young peach wine, thick red but still light,
Fresh grass after frost, green but getting
thick;

Silence, bead curtain, birds coming back,
Birds singing over one spring of sadness.

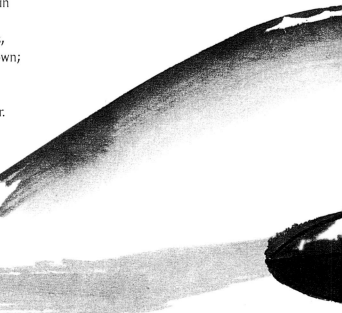

TAKEN from the famed *Jade Prayer Mat*, this poem reflects on the common quality of lust compared to its more elusive counterpart, thought.

Easy to get is the body,
difficult to get is the mind;
easy to pass is the time,
difficult to pass is the trouble.

☯

BECAUSE mandarin ducks usually mate for life, the Chinese use them as symbols of marriage. In ancient China, marital beds were commonly made up with 'mandarin pillows.' These were pillows on which pictures of mandarin ducks had been embroidered.

Quiet chamber, guessing by herself,
mandarin duck, lost companion with no news;
perfume powder, on the arm still has scent,
boxes over the bed are buried in the dust;
beautiful face hollow skims the mirror,
cloudy hair, loose, drops the jade pin;
the horse is not coming, tired eyes,
leave the empty mandarin pillow,
tears over the face.

☯

THIS poem, also from *Jade Prayer Mat*, underscores the importance of sexual balance.

Take it for a long term, Yin and Yang
will be balancing,
take it for too much, water and fire
will be fighting;
take it as medicine, one will enjoy the
opening of the body channel,
take it as a meal, one will suffer the
loss of Chi and blood.

IN this poem from *Jin Ping Mei*, a lover is being told not to worry about life. What will happen, will happen, and in even the most modest of lives there are good times. In the last two verses, the word 'yuan' means 'chance,' and the word 'Xian' is a Taoist word for an earthly or heavenly god or goddess.

Wide character, wide tolerant, years passing by
People born, people die, in front of our eyes;
Following high, following down, following
the fate,
With long, with short, without complaint;
One has, one does not have, there is no
need to worry
A house rich, a house poor, all depends
on the sky;
Food, clothes, one's life going with the yuan
One day you rest, one day you are Xian.

THE READING LIST

Chinese history is rich in erotic literature. The following texts, which are frequently referred to in later writings, discuss the role sex plays in balancing yin and yang:

Biography of Gods and Goddesses
Written c. 1100 B.C., *Biography of Gods and Goddesses* is a book of myths. One is about a king from Western Chou who learned about sexual yin and yang from the Western Kingdom Queen.

Jade Prayer Mat Also called *Carnal Prayer Mat*, this fictional morality tale was written during the Ming dynasty, and admonishes readers against the dangers of wanton sex. The book tells the story of a man named Wei Yang Shen (No End Fellow). In search of the ultimate sexual experience, Wei Yang Shen had a penal implant and began sleeping with other men's wives. In the meantime, his neglected wife went to work in a whorehouse and soon became famous for her lovemaking. When Wei Yang Sheng heard about this prostitute, he went to meet her. But when the prostitute,

his wife, saw him, she hung herself and his lustful search ended in tragedy.

Peng Zu Ching Written c. 2700 B.C., *Peng Zu Ching* is based on the true story of Peng Zu, a man who looked 50 when he was 100 years old. Peng Zu attributed his youthfulness to yin-and-yang-strengthening sex. When the Yellow Emperor heard about Peng Zu, he sent Lady Cai to the old man in order to learn his secrets. This book is about the conversation between Peng Zu and Lady Cai.

Jin Ping Mei A masterpiece of fiction and poetry celebrating sex, *Jin Ping Mei* was written during the Ming dynasty (c. A.D. 1368-1644). The poems tell the story of a wealthy man who married three different women: Jin, Ping, and Mei.

The Mystic Master of the Grotto Written during the Tang dynasty (A.D. 618-906) by either a Taoist, Chang Ting, or the director of the Imperial School of Medicine, Li Tsung-hsuan, this book features graphic descriptions of different types of foreplay and intercourse.

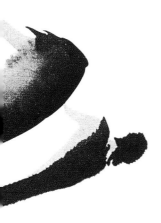

ACCORDING to Taoism, events happen for a reason—even sad events like the departure of a lover. This poem, taken from *Jin Ping Mei*, encourages the reader not to become emotional in the face of what must be. Note that in ancient Chinese, the word 'qian' means 'the ultimate yang,' or 'the ultimate heaven.' The word 'kin' means 'the ultimate yin,' or 'the ultimate earth.'

Going away a thousand miles is not far;
coming back in ten years is not over-long.
Everything should be among the qian and kin;
why worry about leaving and separating.

☯

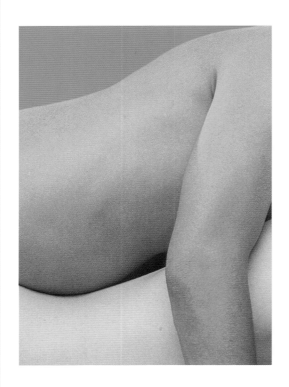

CHAPTER TWO

TRADITIONAL CHINESE RELIGIONS

SEXUAL ENERGY CAN BE
HARNESSED AND CULTIVATED
FOR LONGEVITY, SPIRITUAL
GROWTH, AND HEALING.

TAOISM

BEFORE Taoism was founded in ancient China, shamans lived in harmony with their natural environment, often dwelling in mountain hideaways. They served communities by interpreting omens, predicting weather cycles, and acting as spiritual links between local populations and invisible spirit worlds.

According to legend, shamans could control forces of nature, travel through mountains, and visit the stars. In addition to these mythic abilities, the shamans were responsible for ancient Chinese sciences such as astronomy. They also developed meditation systems and energy circulation exercises. Out of this shamanistic tradition, Taoism was born.

LAOZI

Taoism is attributed to a philosopher named Laozi (also known as Li Erh or Lao Tzu) who lived during the Chou dynasty (c. 580 B.C.). An officer of the royal library, he became enlightened and decided to retreat from society, traveling to far Western China on a water buffalo. Upon reaching a distant mountain pass, the Keeper of the Pass, Wen-Shih, convinced Laozi to record his insights in what became known as the *Tao Te Ching* (also called the *Dao De Jing*). Often called the Tao or Dao (which means 'the way'), the book of philosophy is a kind of manual of meditation and self-transformation.

Laozi was aided by his student, a philosopher named Zhuangzi. They developed a spiritual ideology based on ancient nature worship. A basic tenet of Taoism is the order and harmony of nature, which is considered more stable and enduring than the power of any human government. the creative path of nature—not the values of human society.

Taoist interest in natural medicine advanced knowledge of herbal medicine, including the role diet plays in health (in fact Taoists developed macrobiotic cooking), the importance of movement and massage t strength, and the health-supportive power of sex.

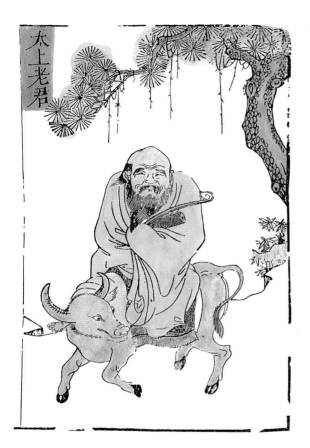

TAOISM'S NINE HEALING ARTS

Taoism emphasized the life-prolonging power of good health using these nine healing arts:

1 Daily Meditation

Daily meditation helps a person stay centered by aligning body, breath, and mind. Meditation is sometimes referred to as Inner Alchemy, or the path to enlightenment and immortality.

2 Nutrition

The Chinese combine food and prescribe diets based on the energetic qualities of food and the specific needs of the individual.

3 Movement Arts

Taoist movement arts include qi gong, tai chi, and martial arts, which are used to train both the physical and energetic bodies. The first three healing arts—meditation, nutrition, and movement arts—are known collectively as the "Three Pillars of Health."

4 Herbal Medicine

According to Chinese herbal medicine, every herb has an energetic quality that can be used to heal a specific symptom or illness.

5 Acupuncture

Acupuncture is the stimulation of specific points along the body with needles. Related to that is acupressure, where the same points are stimulated with finger pressure, herbs, or heat.

6 Feng Shui

Feng Shui is the science of maximizing natural positive energy by strategic placement. It allows people to exist harmoniously with the earth.

7 The Yin and Yang Method

The yin and yang method encourages health and healing through male and female energies, which are exchanged during intercourse.

8 Divination

Divination is the art of seeing and interpreting signs. The ancient Chinese believed that in all things, the microcosm is a mirror of the macrocosm. Thus, a healing system such as reflexology uses one body part to treat a disease of the entire body.

9 Bodywork

Chinese bodywork is used to encourage the efficient flow of energy throughout the body. This bodywork includes various forms of massage and soft tissue manipulation (Tui Na), acupressure (Anmo), and internal organ massage (Chi Nei Tsang).

RELEVANT SELECTIONS FROM THE TAO TE CHING

THE *Tao Te Ching* or *Tao* (which means "the way") is to Taoism what the Bible is to Christianity, the Torah to Judaism and the Koran to Islam—a kind of religious and philosophical guidebook. To become better acquainted with the religion responsible for sexual yin and yang, we offer the following selections from the Tao:

WITHIN Taoism, balance is the ideal state, a state needed for optimal physical and emotional well-being. Thus, the importance of balance is the subject of Chapter 24.

CHAPTER 24
EXCESS

He who stands on his tiptoes does not
stand firm; he who stretches his legs
does not walk (easily). (So), he who displays
himself does not shine;
he who asserts his own views
is not distinguished;
he who vaunts himself does not find
his merit acknowledged; he who is self-
conceited has no superiority
allowed to him. Such conditions,
viewed from the standpoint of the Tao,
are like remnants of food, or a tumor
on the body, which all dislike.
Hence those who pursue (the course)
of the Tao do not adopt and allow them.

TAOISM espouses a certain "theory of relativity" that teaches one can only know a thing by first knowing its opposite. For instance, as Chapter 2 of the Tao states, one cannot know beauty unless first knowing ugliness.

CHAPTER 2
COMPARISONS

All in the world know the beauty
of the beautiful, and in doing
this they have (the idea of) what ugliness is;
they all know the skill
of the skillful, and in doing this they
have (the idea of) what the
want of skill is.

So it is that existence and non-existence
give birth the one to
(the idea of) the other; that difficulty
and ease produce the one (the
idea of) the other; that length and
shortness fashion out the one the
figure of the other; that (the ideas of)
height and lowness arise from

TAOISM 'theory of relativity' that teaches one can only know a thing by first knowing its opposite, also applies to pride. One cannot know glory without humility.

CHAPTER 28
OPPOSITES

Who knows his manhood's strength,
Yet still his female feebleness maintains;
As to one channel flow the many drains,
All come to him, yea, all beneath the sky.
Thus he the constant excellence retains;
The simple child again, free from all stains.

Who knows how white attracts,
Yet always keeps himself within black's shade,
The pattern of humility displayed,
Displayed in view of all beneath the sky;

the contrast of the one with the other;
that the musical notes and
tones become harmonious through the
relation of one with another; and
that being before and behind give the
idea of one following another.

Therefore the sage manages affairs without
doing anything, and
conveys his instructions without
the use of speech.

All things spring up, and there is
not one which declines to show
itself; they grow, and there is no claim
made for their ownership;
they go through their processes, and
there is no expectation (of a
reward for the results). The work is
accomplished, and there is no
resting in it (as an achievement).

The work is done, but how no one can see;
'Tis this that makes the power not cease to be.

He in the unchanging excellence arrayed,
Endless return to man's first state has made.
Who knows how glory shines,
Yet loves disgrace, nor e'er for it is pale;
Behold his presence in a spacious vale,
To which men come from all beneath the sky.
The unchanging excellence completes its tale;
The simple infant man in him we hail.

The unwrought material, when divided
and distributed, forms
vessels. The sage, when employed, becomes
the Head of all the
Officers (of government);
and in his greatest regulations he
employsno violent measures.

WHEN using sex as a healing tool, it is important
to realize that there are times when orgasm
should be withheld. Chapter 12 explains how
repressing one's desires can be beneficial.

CHAPTER 12
RESTRAINT
Color's five hues from th' eyes
their sight will take;
Music's five notes the ears as deaf can make;
The flavors five deprive the mouth of taste;
The chariot course, and the wild hunting waste
Make mad the mind;
and objects rare and strange,
Sought for, men's conduct will to evil change.

Therefore the sage seeks to satisfy (the craving
of) the belly, and not
the (insatiable longing of the) eyes.
He puts from him the latter,
and prefers to seek the former.

CHAPTER 71 acknowledges the importance of
recognizing personal limitations, a particularly
Taoist thought that can be seen in the sexual
exercises found in this book.

CHAPTER 71
LIMITATION
To know and yet (think) we do not know
is the highest (attainment);
not to know (and yet think) we do know
is a disease.

It is simply by being pained at
(the thought of) having this disease
that we are preserved from it.
The sage has not the disease.
He knows the pain that would be inseparable
from it, and therefore
hedoes not have it.

CONFUCIANISM

CONFUCIANISM was started by Chiu Kong (c. 551-479 B.C.), who was also called Kong the Philosopher, or K'ung Fu-tse. Confucius, as he is known today, was born in the feudal state of Lu, in modern Shangdong province. He emphasized the importance of *li* (proper behavior), *jen* (sympathetic attitude), and *xiao* (ancestor worship)—all tenets that remain important in modern China.

Confucius's audience was largely limited to the aristocrats for whom he worked. At age 19 he entered the service of a noble family as superintendent of parks and herds. When he was 32 he was asked to teach ancient rituals to a minister's sons. At age 33 he went to Lo-yang, the imperial capital, to study the customs and traditions of the Chou Empire, which had split into numerous warring states of various sizes, leaving the capital to function solely as a religious center. On this occasion Confucius is said to have visited Laozi, the founder of Taoism. When Confucius was 34 years old, the prince of Lu was forced to flee, threatened by powerful rivals among the local nobility. Confucius accompanied him to a neighboring state. At the age of 51 he returned to political life, working as minister of justice and finally prime minister of Lu.

Considering Confucius's long-standing association with the aristocracy, it is no surprise that his philosophy first became popular among the ruling and scholarly elite. While Confucianism began circulating among these classes during the Han dynasty (207 B.C-A.D. 220), it wasn't until the Song dynasty (A.D. 960-1278) that it became the unofficial state religion. It was during this time that the doctrine grew into a system for the training of officials, and public schools were replaced with Confucian schools.

While Confucianism and the previously popular Taoism diverged on many points, the two religions disagreed most strongly on the role of women.

Taoism celebrated feminine strength and declared it an integral part of well-being, prescribing romance and sex as a way for women to achieve stronger feminine (yin) energy. Confucius himself, however, spoke disparagingly of women, remarking frequently that nothing is so hard to handle as a female and a little man. Furthermore, he was contemptuous of romance and insisted on the segregation of women. This particular element of Confucianism was largely responsible for the sexually repressed climate and oppression of women that marks China's later dynasties.

The Three Gang, which means major principle, promoted social structure through a three-tiered hierarchy: The Gang of the emperor and follower; the Gang of father and son; and the Gang of husband and wife. It meant that the followers must listen to the emperor; the son must listen to the father; and the wife must listen to the husband.

PEACEFUL COEXISTANCE

Since its beginning, Confucianism bacame intertwined with Taoism. Laozi (Lao Tzu), the founder of Taoism, is often regarded as one of Confucius's early mentors. And while the Confucian tradition served as the ethical and religious foundation of many ancient Chinese institutions, elements of Taoism—such as qi gong, herbal medicine, and views of yin and yang—offered a range of alternatives and embellishments to Confucian beliefs. For the majority of Chinese, there was no choosing between Confucianism and Taoism. Other than a few strict Confucians and a few strict Taoists, the vast majority of Chinese subscribed to elements of both religions.

CONFUCIUS SAY

Confucius was well known for his teaching style, which revolved around short fables and one- or two-sentence proclamations. Although Confucianism has declined in importance in China since the Communist Revolution, its estimated five million followers can find spiritual lessons in the *Book of Analects* (*Lun Yu*), from which the following bits of wisdom are collected:

■ Sorrow not because men do not know you; but sorrow that you do not know men.

■ When you know a thing, maintain you know it; when you do not, acknowledge it. This is the characteristic of knowledge.

■ To see what is right and not to do it, that is cowardice.

■ The superior man is not contentious. He contends only as in competitions of archery; and when he wins he will present his cup to his competitor.

■ He who has sinned against Heaven has none other to whom his prayer may be addressed.

■ Tell me, is there anyone who is able for one whole day to apply the energy of his mind to virtue? It may be that there are such, but I have never met with one.

■ The scholar who is intent upon learning the truth, yet is ashamed of his poor clothes and food, is not worthy to be discoursed with.

■ It is as hard to be poor without complaining as to be rich without becoming arrogant.

■ The superior men are sparing in their words and profuse in their deeds.

■ Confucius was asked, "What say you of the remark, 'Repay enmity with kindness'?" And he replied, "How then would you repay kindness? Repay kindness with kindness, and enmity with justice."

■ I have not yet met the man who loves virtue as he loves beauty.

■ Not to react after committing an error is in itself an error.

■ Three things the superior man guards against: lust of the flesh in youth, combativeness in maturity, and ambition in old age.

■ Confucius was asked, "What say you are the essentials of good government?" He answered, "The ruler should esteem the five excellences and avoid the four evils.

The five excellences are:
• plenitude without extravagance;
• taxation without exciting discontent;
• desire without covetousness;
• dignity without haughtiness;
• majesty without fierceness.
The four evils to be avoided are:
• without instruction in the law, to inflict punishment—that is tyranny;
• without proper warning to expect perfect adherence—that is oppression;
• late in giving orders and expecting early obedience—that is robbery;
• to tax and to spend in a stingy manner—that is a misuse of government function."

BUDDHISM

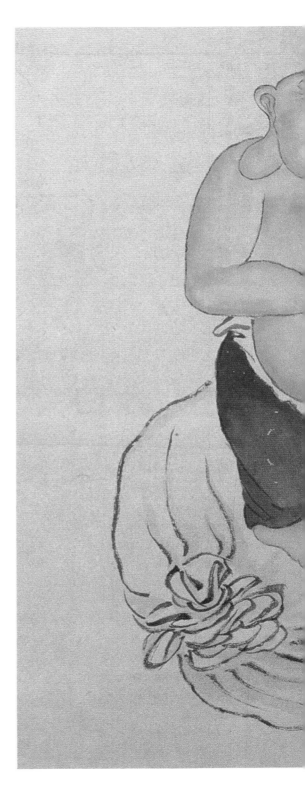

THOUGH Buddhism played an important role in ancient China, it was actually founded in Northern India in the sixth century B.C. by Siddhartha Gautama, who became known as the Buddha (Enlightened One). The Buddha achieved enlightenment (Nirvana) through meditation, and established a community of monks to follow his example and encourage others. Buddhism teaches that Nirvana can be reached through meditation and good moral and religious behavior. It also maintains that people are reincarnated and that their lives are happy or sad depending on their actions (karma) in a previous life. Buddhist belief is centered around the Four Noble Truths: all living beings must suffer; desire and self-importance cause suffering; the achievement of Nirvana ends suffering; and Nirvana can be attained through meditation and righteous actions, thoughts, and attitudes.

Unlike Confucius, Buddha preached respect, love, and eternal salvation for not only men but for women, gods, and animals. Buddhist monks were commanded not to harm any living reature—the reason vegetarianism is so strongly associated with Buddhism. Buddhism encourages four modes of inner conduct: loving-kindness, ompassion, sympathetic joy, and equanimity toward the impure and evil.

While there are many types of Buddhism, Zen Buddhism is the most prevalent in China. In fact, the name 'Zen' is derived from the Chinese Chan'an-na, which is a corruption of the Buddhist Dhyana, meaning 'meditation.' According to legend, Buddhism was brought to China in the late fifth century A.D. by an Indian monk named Bodhidharma. It did not become popular until nearly a century later, when Hui-neng, a Chinese Taoist philosopher and theologian, established Zen as a sect of Buddhism.

In India, Buddhism incorporated the idea of tantric practice as the art of lovemaking.

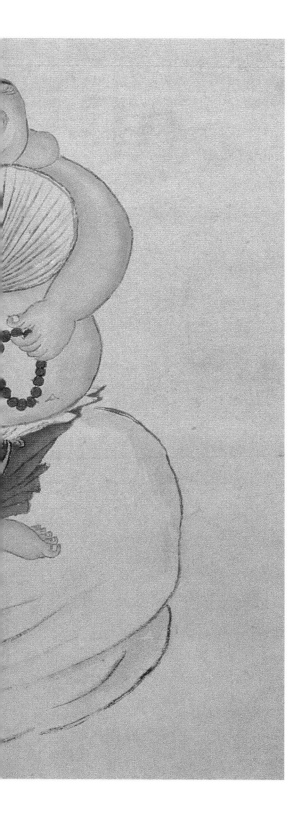

THE BUDDHIST WAY

Like Taoism's *Tao* and Confucianism's *Book of Analects*, Buddhism's *Dhamapada* is a text of religious wisdom designed to help followers practice and maintain their faith. Composed of short proverbs, the *Dhamapada* offers easy-to-understand lessons. Here are a few selections:

■ All that we are is the result of what we have thought: It is founded on our thoughts and is made up of our thoughts.

■ As rain breaks through an ill-thatched roof, so lust breaks through the ill-trained mind.

■ Like a beautiful flower full of color but without scent are the fair words of him who himself does not act accordingly.

■ As a solid rock is not shaken by the wind, so the wise man does not waver before blame or praise.

■ An evil deed, like freshly drawn milk, does not turn sour at once.

■ There is an old saying: They blame him who sits silent; they blame him who speaks much; they blame him who says little. There is no one in the world who does not get blamed.

■ Life is easy to live for a man who is without shame, bold as a crow, a mischief-maker, insulting, arrogant, and dissolute. But life is hard to live for a man who is modest, always looking for what is pure, free from attachment, unassuming, and clear of vision.

■ All men tremble at punishment and all men fear death; remember that you are like them and do not kill nor cause slaughter.

SEXUAL
YIN &
YANG:
THE
BASICS

CHAPTER THREE

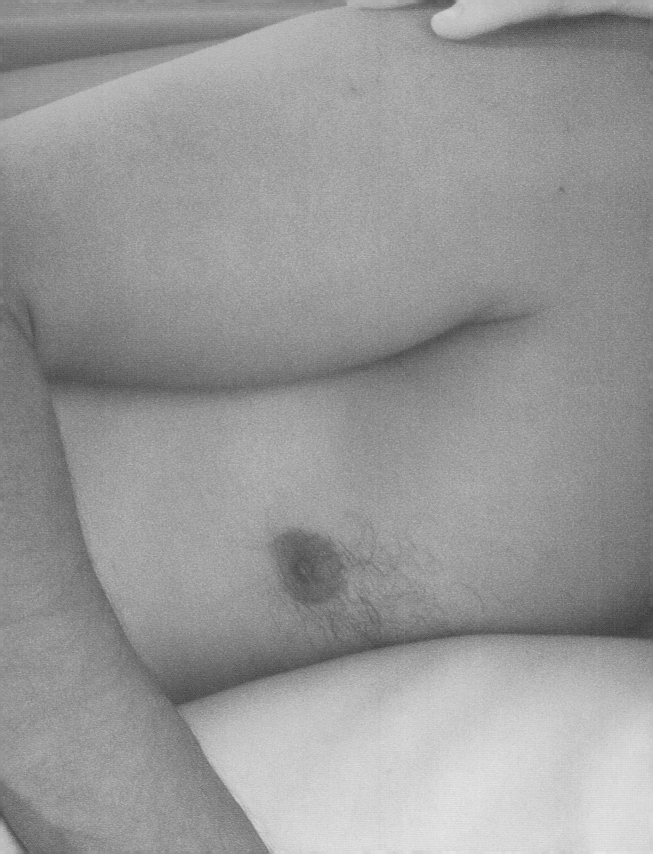

EXPLORING SEXUAL YIN & YANG

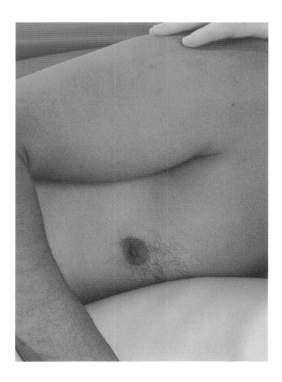

YIN AND YANG IS A PARTICULARLY CHINESE CONCEPT, ONE THAT DENOTES THE TWO OPPOSING FORCES THAT EXIST WITHIN EVERY LIVING THING.

ABOUT YIN & YANG

WHILE yin and yang is often explained simply as contrary energies, the principle is actually more complex: Everything contains and is balanced by its own mutually dependent polar opposites. The concept is symbolized by the sun and the moon—the two opposing forces active over the earth—and is often depicted as a two-toned circle. Within the dark half of the circle there is a small light dot, and within the light half lies a small dark dot. This suggests that, though opposites, there is a necessary relationship between yin and yang. Neither exists in and of itself. There is also the meaning of the words 'yin' and 'yang.' In addition to 'the moon,' yin alternatively means 'the dark side of a mountain,' while yang means both 'the sun' and 'the light side of a mountain.'

THIS AND THAT

In China, it is common to attribute various personality traits, weather patterns, health conditions, and other states to either yin or yang.

YIN	YANG
Female	Male
Earth	Heaven
Moon	Sun
Conservation	Destruction
Absorbing	Reflecting
Winter	Summer
Receptive	Ejecting
Dark	Bright
Even	Uneven
Soft	Hard
Calm	Movement
Sorrow	Elation
Mental strength	Physical strength

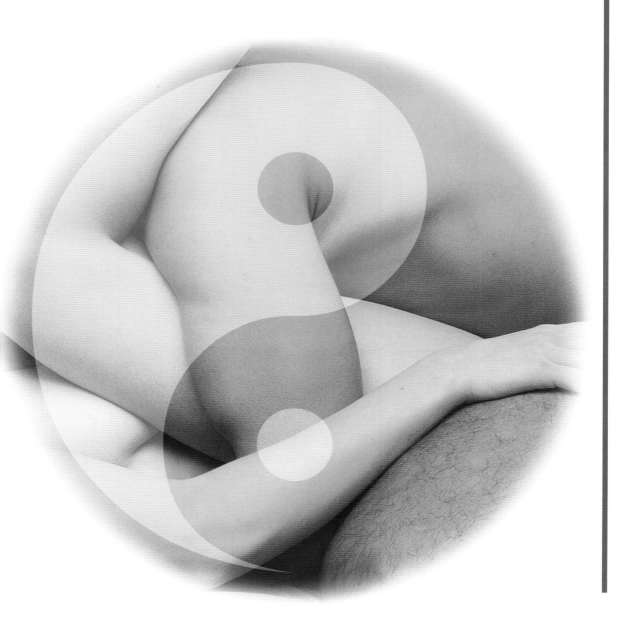

While the concept may have been in China much longer, the term 'yin and yang' wasn't created until late in the Zhou dynasty (1027-256 B.C.), when philosophers were seeking to describe the way opposites depended on each other: There can be no light without darkness, nor life without death. According to these ancient philosophers, yin and yang is an ever-changing combination. Day gives way to night, something hot can grow cold, someone outgoing can become self-protective, the living eventually die. According to Chinese thought, this constant flux is a good thing. It is what creates chi, the life-giving force of the universe.

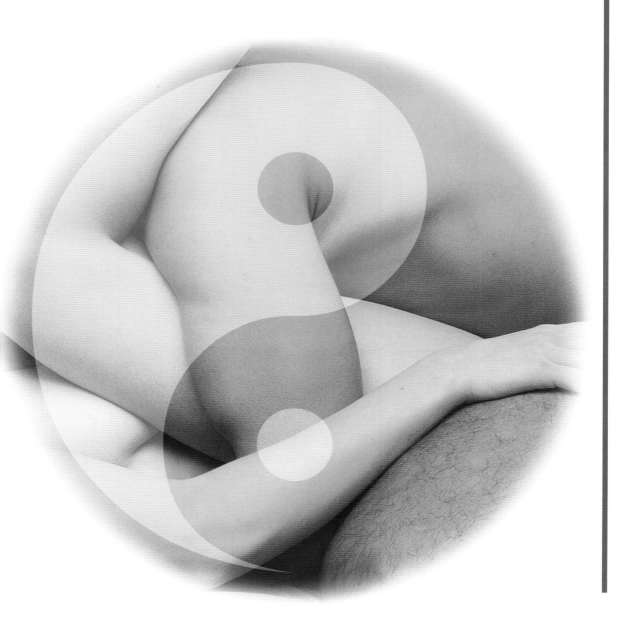

Perhaps nowhere is the concept of yin and yang so well-known to Westerners as in Chinese medicine. As previously discussed, one of the best-known and earliest Chinese medical texts is *The Yellow Emperor's Classic of Internal Medicine*, believed to have been written during the third millennium B.C. by the mythical Yellow Emperor.

Besides general theory, the book discusses natural drugs, gymnastics, and minor surgery.

Many of the concepts presented in *The Yellow Emperor's Classic* have become well-established elements of modern Chinese medicine. The most central of these is the maintenance of balance. Ideally, the human body should be in a perfectly

THE FIVE ELEMENTS

While yin and yang may be the pillar of Chinese medicine, the five elements (also called the five phases) established by the Yellow Emperor also play a role. These elements roughly correspond to the five geographic regions found in ancient China, which also reflect human organs and other physical features.

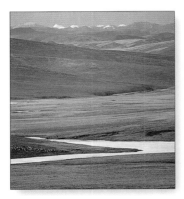

Central: neutral temperature, earth, yellow soil

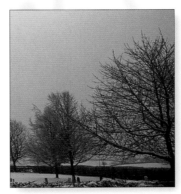

North: very cold, winter, water, black soil

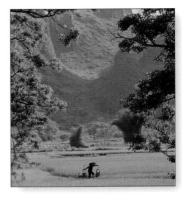

East: warm, spring, wood, green soil

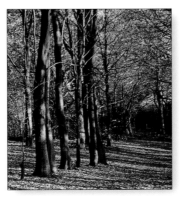

West: cool, fall, metal, white soil

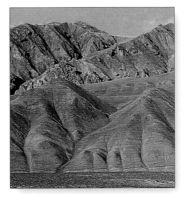

South: very hot, summer, fire, red soil

equalized state. Activity should match rest, food intake should match calorie expenditure, and so on. According to the Yellow Emperor's book, illness is caused by an imbalance of yin and yang due to intense emotion, activity, temperature, or other influences. Curing an illness thus depends on accurately finding the source of the imbalance. However, because the body's organs and systems are interrelated, diagnosing such an imbalance can be tricky. For example, because it is solid, the liver is considered a yin organ. But the liver also promotes the flow of energy, which is a yang quality.

Acupuncture, herbal treatments, qi gong, sexual yin and yang—all are health-supportive measures used within Chinese medicine to maintain or create a balance between yin and yang. When yin and yang are brought into balance, illness is diminished and well-being and vitality are increased.

TYPES OF IMBALANCE

There are many varieties of imbalance between yin and yang. When trying to decide what type of disparity is present, doctors of Chinese medicine look for the following clues:

Too much yin Characterized by cold symptoms, including joint problems, bone conditions, and kidney disorders.

Too much yang Characterized by heat symptoms, including circulation conditions, heart problems, and fevers.

Too little yin Characterized by internal heat symptoms, including skin conditions, and by lowered ability to tolerate physical or emotional stress.

Too little yang Characterized by general coldness, including fatigue, general weakness, and incontinence.

ADVICE FROM THE YELLOW EMPEROR'S CLASSIC OF MEDICINE

'If Yang is overly powerful, then Yin may be too weak. If Yin is particularly strong, then Yang is apt to be defective. If the male force is overwhelming, then there will be excessive heat. If the female force is overwhelming, then there will be excessive cold. Exposure to repeated and severe heat will induce chills. Cold injures the body while heat injures the spirit. When the spirit is hurt, severe pain will ensue. When the body is hurt, there will be swelling. Thus, when severe pain occurs first and swelling comes on later, one may infer that a disharmony in the spirit has done harm to the body. Likewise, when swelling appears first and severe pain is felt later on, one can say that a dysfunction in the body has injured the spirit. Nature has four seasons and five elements. To grant long life, these seasons and elements must store up the power of creation in cold, heat, dryness, moisture, and wind. Man has five viscera in which these five climates are transformed into joy, anger, sympathy, grief, and fear. The emotions of joy and anger are injurious to the spirit just as cold and heat are injurious to the body. Violent anger depletes Yin; violent joy depletes Yang. When rebellious emotions rise to Heaven, the pulse expires and leaves the body. When joy and anger are without moderation, then cold and heat exceed all measure, and life is no longer secure. Yin and Yang should be respected to an equal extent.'

SITUATIONS TO AVOID

ANCIENT Chinese healers believed that in order to maintain overall wellness and avoid illness, there were times when one should refrain from sex. These temporary bouts of celibacy were thought to preserve the balance of chi within the body. Pronounced 'chee' and alternately called 'vital energy,' 'primal energy,' and 'the life force,' chi is the fundamental energy found in all living things. For good health, peace of mind, and even conception, this energy must circulate unimpeded throughout the body. Yet severe weather, various physical conditions, and some mental states disrupt the steady flow of this important energy within the body. Fortunately for those interested in the connection between intercourse and health, a number of China's healers created sexual guidelines detailing when to refrain from intimacy. Extremely specific, these instructions encompass a range of situations, including specific weather patterns, emotions, indoor and outdoor locations, times of day, and a range of bodily states.

Following are some of these guidelines, which fall into three categories:

■ Three Forbidden Situations
■ Seven Body Conditions
■ Five Types of Tiredness.

THREE FORBIDDEN SITUATIONS

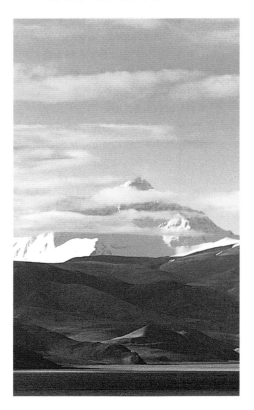

According to Chinese healing beliefs, making love during Forbidden Situations can disrupt the even flow of chi, causing the energy to stagnate in specific areas of the body. This makes it difficult to exchange chi with your partner. It also weakens health, causes illness, and can even threaten the safety of an unborn child. Forbidden Situations include the following three specific circumstances during which sex should be avoided:

■ Heaven Forbidden
■ Human Forbidden
■ Earth Forbidden

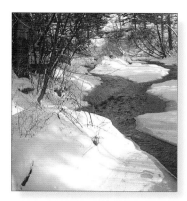

GREAT COLD
Temperatures lower than 15°F
(-9°C)

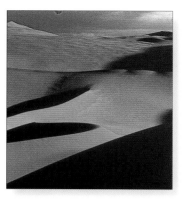

GREAT HEAT
Temperatures higher than 90°F
(32°C)

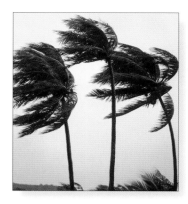

GREAT WINDS
Speeds of 35 or more miles
per hour

HEAVEN FORBIDDEN

Western healing traditions rarely link weather, sex, and health. In China, however, the three elements are intimately entwined by chi. Severe weather conditions affect the earth's magnetic and energy fields, which in turn disrupt the constant flow of health-supportive chi within the body. For this reason, sex and other chi-boosting activities, such as tai chi and qi gong, are discouraged during certain weather conditions. Severe weather is also believed to impede conception.

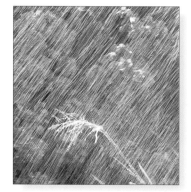

GREAT RAINS
Rainfall of 2 or more inches
per hour

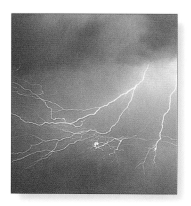

THUNDERSTORMS
Any storm with audible thunder

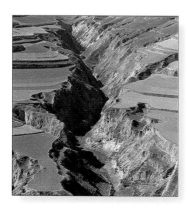

EARTHQUAKES
A quake measuring 2 or higher on
the Richter scale

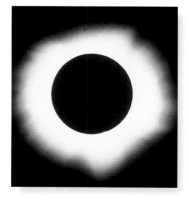

ECLIPSES
Any partial or full solar or lunar
eclipse

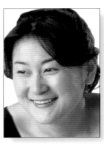

INTENSELY HAPPY
Western cultures view joy as positive—unconnected to danger. In Eastern cultures, extreme joy is something to be cautious of. Chinese healers believe that intercourse during this time can stress the heart as well as taxe the kidneys by sending an overabundance of chi flooding through the body.

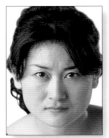

ANGRY
Anger is a distracting emotion that can divert one's attention from intimacy. Because it is closely associated with violence, anger may impair one's physical judgement and can lessen one's concern for his or her partner. Taoists further believe that having intercourse while angry can lead to central nervous system dysfunction.

INTOXICATED
Chinese healers believe that having sex while under the influence of alcohol or a drug causes irregular chi within the body. This in turn can lead to a decrease in general well-being, lowered immunity, and fatigue. Whether overly inebriated from alcohol, prescription medication, or recreational drugs, the resulting loss of physical and mental control can also impair sexual judgement and limit sexual functioning.

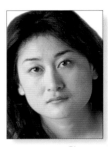

SAD
Sadness saps energy, causing weakness and lethargy—conditions made even worse by the rigors of intercourse. Chinese healers believe that the lungs in particular suffer when sad individuals have sex. The result is a persistent cough and increased general fatigue.

HUMAN FORBIDDEN

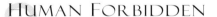

According to Taoist tradition, intense physical and emotional states cause irregularities in the chi that courses through the body. Because sex intensifies chi, intercourse should be avoided during these circumstances. Intense physical and emotional factors can also distract you, making it difficult to give lovemaking and your partner the attention they deserve.

NOTE: For the Western reader, abstaining during some of these conditions makes great sense—such as avoiding sex when drunk, for instance. Other suggestions—such as avoiding intimacy during times of great joy—are uniquely Eastern.

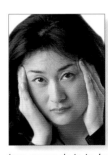

WORRIED For many people, worry is often physically manifested in a nervous stomach, an ache illustrated by the saying 'my stomach is in knots.' Taoists similarly believe that worry is linked to stomach conditions; having sex while worried causes chi to leach from the rest of the body and drain into the abdomen.

FULL FROM EATING If the stomach is at least 70 percent full, it is better to wait before having sex. After eating, blood rushes to the stomach and the body expends its energy on digestion. This is why Chinese healers advise refraining from all activity after meals, including school work, washing hair, and cleaning. Because undigested food may weigh against lower body parts, intercourse on a full stomach can lead to discomfort and pain.

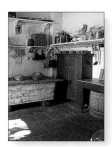

KITCHEN
Food in ancient China was scarce. To ensure food for their families, the Chinese worshipped a god named Zao Wang Ye, meaning 'King of the Oven'. This god resided in the kitchen. Doing anything to disrespect him—having sex in his space, for instance—could disrupt the chi running within a person's body and lead to impaired health

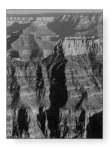

MAJOR GEOGRAPHIC FEATURE
The Grand Canyon, the Mississippi River, and the painted deserts are all major geographic features. Just as many Native American's believe these areas attract both spirits and energy, so do the Chinese. Having sex in such powerful areas can greatly disrupt the body's flow of chi, leaving an individual fatigued and susceptible to illness.

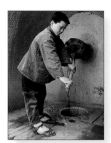

WELL
Today, we turn on a faucet and out comes a steady stream of water; yet, most of us are so removed from the source of our water that we have no idea where it originates. There was a time when everyone in a town knew where their water came from—a shared well. Because this water source was so precious to so many, it was imperative that nothing be done to harm it. In ancient China, people were not allowed to dip their bare hands into a well, nor were they allowed to have sex near one for fear that it might become contaminated, thus polluting the water for an entire population. Since any action that brings hardship to others—in this case, dirtying their water—is believed to damage a person's flow of chi, it became an important Taoist principle not to have sex near a water source.

EARTH FORBIDDEN

In China, all physical things are thought to radiate energy. Ancient Taoists were especially sensitive to natural landmarks, creating detailed rules for constructing homes, temples, tombs, wells, and other buildings in spiritual harmony with their surroundings. If this harmony is achieved, then the spirits will look kindly on the family and descendants.

The Chinese believe that where you do something is as important as where you put something. Because natural and human-built structures have chi-altering properties, where you make love can affect your health and mental wellness. According to Chinese beliefs, having sex in these forbidden locations may not have an immediate health effect but it can hurt one's fate—specifically, it may bring harm to one's descendants.

EARLY TAOIST EDICT

'Ejaculation is strictly forbidden when a man is drunk or gorged with food. Such emissions injure a man a hundred times more than under normal conditions and may cause dizziness and ugly sores.'

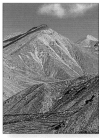

MOUNTAIN
In China, mountains are considered intensely holy places where spirits and gods reside. Having sex in such a sacred environment is an act of irreverence that can damage a person's chi, which in turn can lead to lowered immunity, general fatigue, and ill health.

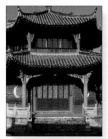

PLACE OF WORSHIP
Churches, temples, synagogues, monasteries, and other houses of worship are sacred. Having sex in holy sites is highly disrespectful and can disrupt the even circulation of health-supportive chi within the body.

SEVEN BODY CONDITIONS

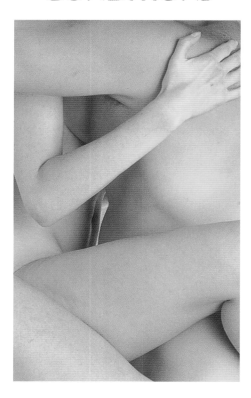

In ancient China, there were many experts on the art of the bedchamber. In addition to the Taoists, Lady Su (c. 3000 B.C.), was a kind of sex therapist so famous for her knowledge that she was said to regularly advise rulers.

According to Lady Su, there were specific instances when making love could harm one's health. Many of her suggestions were later adopted by Taoists, explaining the overlap between her recommendations and those given by Chinese healers.

DREAM DOCTOR

Ancient Chinese healers regularly used dreams to diagnose problems of the inner organs. The following dream diagnoses are based on excerpts from an ancient medical text, *Yellow Inner Bible*:

■ Dreams of fighting, killing an animal, or using a metal weapon in some other capacity: a lung condition. According to the Chinese Five Element theory, lung problems are 'metal' disorders.

■ Dreams of drowning, swimming, or otherwise being in water: a kidney condition. According to the Chinese Five Element theory, kidney problems are 'water' disorders.

■ Dreams of forests, trees, grass, flowers, or plants: a liver condition. According to the Chinese Five Element theory, liver problems are 'wood' disorders.

■ Dreams of fire, cooking, fireplaces, a burning house, or a forest fire: a heart condition. According to the Chinese Five Element theory, heart problems are 'fire' disorders.

■ Dreams of dirt, soil, mud, sowing seeds, bricks, or of starving: an illness affecting the spleen. According to the Chinese Five Element theory, spleen problems are 'earth' disorders.

MOON OR SUN NOT CLEAR

There are times when a planet wholly or partially obstructs the view of either the sun or moon. Other times, an eclipse may block the sun or moon from sight. Regardless, when an element of the solar system changes alignment, it disrupts the earth's chi. To have sex when the sun or moon is not clearly visible can create chaotic, uneven movement of chi within the body. Sex during this time is especially discouraged for those trying to conceive.

UNCOMFORTABLE SETTING

Comfort is subjective. What is comfortable to one person might be anxiety-provoking for another. Such a situation promotes an even flow of chi between lovers. Usually, however, comfortable describes a private, indoor setting that is free from children, other people, drafts, dirt, disturbances, and anything unpredictable. Any upset to either member of the couple can hinder the flow of chi.

IMMEDIATELY AFTER EATING

After eating, the body's chi congregates in the stomach to aid digestion. Waiting at least 30 minutes after meals before having sex will give the chi a chance to return to its normal flow in the body.

IMMEDIATELY AFTER USING THE TOILET

In a normal waking state, chi flows evenly throughout the body, circulating constantly among the skin, nerves, muscles, bones, and internal organs. The flow of chi into the kidneys, however, is at its

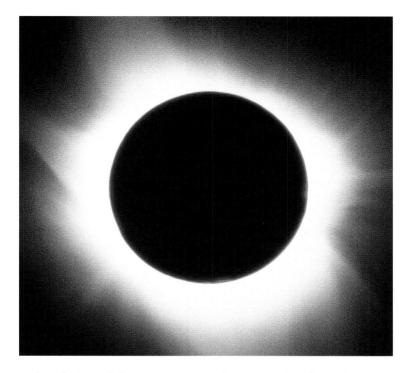

weakest during and after using the bathroom. Having intercourse directly after relieving oneself can further lower the chi in the kidneys and lead to kidney problems. It is important to wait 30 minutes after using the toilet before having sex. This allows the free-flowing chi to make its way back to the kidneys.

WITH WET HAIR

When your hair is wet, chi travels to the head to help preserve precious body heat. This leaves the rest of the body with weak chi. Having sex during this time can leave a person feeling weak, lightheaded, or headachy.

SEVERE WEATHER

Thunderstorms, heavy rains, droughts, snowstorms, hail, typhoons, hurricanes — any type of severe weather affects the earth's chi. Making love during these times can stop the smooth stream of bodily chi, causing it to stagnate in one of the internal organs.

AFTER INTENSE PHYSICAL LABOR

Intense physical activity—whether manual labor or exercise—weakens the body and its chi. After exerting oneself, it is important to wait two or more hours before engaging in another physically demanding pursuit, such as sex. Waiting gives the body time to recover and allows one's chi to rejuvenate.

FIVE TYPES OF TIRED

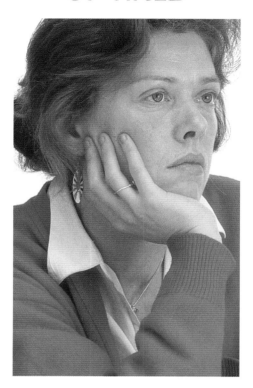

The Five Types of Tiredness is a Taoist theory that describes different levels of fatigue. Although not considered actual illnesses, each of the Five Types of Tiredness is a visible sign that an illness could potentially occur within the body. Tiredness of the Skin is the most superficial variety of tiredness and represents an illness of minor severity. The deeper the fatigue — muscles, ligaments, tendons, bones, blood — the more life-threatening the underlying illness. When experiencing any of the Five Types of Tiredness, Taoist healers prescribe avoiding orgasm as a way of conserving and even building health-supportive chi (for more detailed information on climax-free sex, see 'Why Resist Orgasm' on page 158).

LEVELS OF ILLNESS

The Taoist doctor who perfected the theory of chi was named Bian Que (pronounced 'choi'). Legend holds that around the year 500 B.C., Bian Que observed that by holding his hand over a person's body he could feel subtle vibrations. Areas with irregular vibrations were often damaged organs that were not allowing an even flow of chi.

One day Bian Que is reported to have seen the king of Qi. 'Your majesty, you have illness in your skin,' Bian Que said to the ruler. 'If you don't cure it right now, it will get worse.' 'You must be joking,' said the king. 'I feel fine.'

The second time Bian Que saw the king, he said, 'Your majesty, the illness has traveled to your muscle. If you don't cure it right now, it will get worse.' 'I'm alright,' the king said. 'I will take care of myself.'

Soon thereafter Bian Que was called to the palace. The king was ill and needed Bian Que's help. 'Your majesty,' said Bian Que. 'Your illness has moved past the bone into the marrow, blood, bodily fluid, and nervous system chi. It is too late to do anything.'

Shortly after that last visit, the king died.

THE SKIN

You feel a bit tired. When you look in the mirror, your skin appears pale and perhaps a bit dry. But other than that, you feel fine. Sound familiar? This type of fatigue, called Tired in the Skin, is a symptom of stress, a mild nutritional imbalance, or lack of sleep. Though not life-threatening, these conditions can affect the flow of chi and can make it difficult to conceive. Before having sex, spend one or two days eating well, getting enough rest, and practicing stress-control measures such as deep breathing or meditation.

THE MUSCLES

Anyone who knows what sore, tired muscles feel like knows the symptom called Tired in the Muscle. At this level of fatigue, the muscles feel weak and overtaxed. You may have difficulty carrying any amount of weight and you may suddenly become clumsy. Tired in the Muscles usually occurs with an illness of mild to moderate severity, such as a flu. Having orgasm during such a time can further weaken an already-weakened flow of chi. A better alternative is to see a doctor, eat well and get plenty of rest. Stretching and massage can ease sore muscles.

THE BONES

Americans often use the expression 'bone-tired' to describe the sensation of being physically tired to their bone marrow. The Chinese see Tiredness of the Bones as a symptom of a serious disease, one that may actually involve the bone, such as osteoporosis, or another type of ailment that is quite serious, such as prostate cancer. Because the flow of chi is severely interrupted at this time, orgasm should be avoided. An individual who experiences Tiredness of the Bones should also seek medical care. Doctors of Chinese medicine prescribe calcium-rich foods such as sea vegetables and tofo.

THE LIGAMENTS AND TENDONS

The ligaments connect bones together. The tendons fuse muscles to bone. The Chinese believe that Tiredness of the Ligaments and Tendons is a symptom for a moderate internal illness, such as bronchitis or a bladder infection. An illness of this type causes the chi to weaken before reaching the ligaments, leaving one more susceptible to sprains and overextended joints. An individual who experiences Tiredness of the Ligaments and Tendons should see a doctor and avoid orgasm until he or she recovers. Meanwhile, to ease the chance of muscle sprains, stretching and twisting exercises can be used. These include gymnastics, qi gong, tai chi, or simple at-home movements.

THE MARROW, BODILY FLUID, AND NERVOUS SYSTEM CHI

The Chinese believe that bodily fluids—including blood and bone marrow—are the active components of a body, while the more solid organs and bones are the passive elements. The marrow, bodily fluid, and nervous system are where chi resides. When someone develops Tiredness of the Marrow, Bodily Fluid, and Nervous System Chi, it is a sign that something could be seriously wrong, even life-threatening. This may be a stroke, advanced cancer, leukemia, severe anemia, extensive cholesterol deposits in the arteries, or any other grave illness. Signs include exhaustion, immobility, pallor, and an inelastic quality to the skin. At this point, it is imperative to consult a physician. In China, seafood,

sea vegetables, soy, and nuts are routinely prescribed to strengthen the marrow, bodily fluid, and nervous system chi.

TAKE TIME TO HEAL

The Chinese say that torn ligaments and fractured bones need 100 days to heal.

FAVORABLE SITUATIONS

WAITING until just the right moment to have sex—although the very idea seems foreign in Western cultures—is a common concept in China. Just as there are times, places, and conditions when refraining from sex is best, so are there times, places, and conditions that are ideal for sex. These situations are favored by Taoist healers because they encourage a strong, even flow of chi throughout the body. Having sex in any one of these circumstances is believed to boost immunity, create greater well-being, and help cure existing illnesses.

MAY DAYS

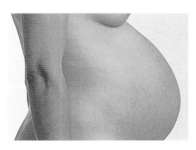

In nature, a large number of animals mate in the spring. Noticing this, doctors in ancient China prescribed spring as the most beneficial time for humans to conceive. May was seen as a particularly healthful month to become pregnant, as this allows a woman to enter her third month in August. This is important for proper brain development. Chinese doctors believe a fetus needs an especially concentrated supply of nutrition during its third month. August is when much of the harvest starts in China, meaning a large supply of fresh, nutritious food for mother and child.

ENVIRONMENTAL

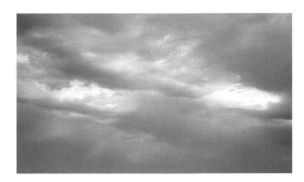

COMFORTABLE INTERIOR SPACE

Indoor sex is the ideal, according to Taoist healers. An indoor location offers privacy and protects a couple from distractions that can block chi and make sex less enjoyable. These distractions include natural elements, animals, insects, and other humans.

NICE WEATHER CONDITIONS

When indoors, it is easy to ignore what is going on outside. However, the weather can affect lovemaking. That's because severe weather conditions—such as a thunderstorm, heavy rain, strong wind, hurricane, and so on—make the earth's chi erratic. Having sex during such a time can block a person's chi as well.

UNOBSTRUCTED CONDITIONS FROM THE EARTH TO THE SUN

The chi that flows over the earth moves most freely when the sun is not blocked by clouds, the moon, or another planet. During eclipses and other astronomical situations that obstruct the sun, it is best to avoid sex. Intercourse during this time can lead to blockages in chi.

HUMAN

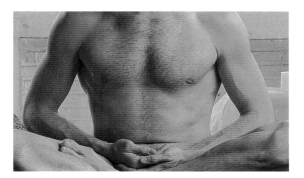

TIMING

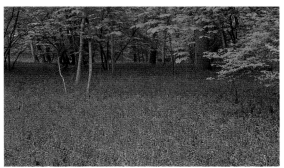

HEALTHY BODY CONDITIONS

Although intercourse is most pleasurable when both partners are physically healthy, an ill individual doesn't have to forego sex entirely. According to Taoists healers, he or she should forego chi-disrupting orgasm—this means lots of foreplay (see 'Healing by the Lover' beginning on page 130).

STABLE EMOTIONAL STATE

In China, a stable emotional state is one that doesn't veer too far from the emotional middle road. Too much happiness is as chi-blocking as too much sadness or anger or worry or any other sentiment. For this reason, the most chi-boosting sex occurs when both partners are feeling calm and neutral.

GOOD TIME OF DAY

Ancient Chinese healers felt that sex during the evening was the most healthful from a chi-boosting point of view. During the early evening, the day's physical work is behind you, and you are relaxed and able to focus on the demands of intercourse— all of which contribute to calm, chi-enhancing sex.

SEASONAL FACTORS

Very few people are willing to wait for a specific season to make love, which is fine. When ancient healers spoke of good seasons for sex, they were speaking strictly in terms of conception. Spring was proposed as the best time to become pregnant, followed by fall, summer, and then winter.

YIN & YANG: ANCIENT WISDOM

The Yellow Emperor, wishing to know more about the art of the bedchamber, learned about yin and yang from Lady Su. Wanting to know more, the Yellow Emperor approached Lady Xuan. 'Lady Su already told me something about Yin and Yang,' said the Yellow Emperor to Lady Xuan. 'But I would like to know more. I am here to listen to your advice.'

'Everything in the universe is made from Yin and Yang elements,' said Lady Xuan. 'Yang will settle by Yin, and Yin will grow by Yang. One Yin and one Yang integrate and move together. So a man will become excited and expand his jade stalk for a woman, and a woman will become excited and open her jade door for a man. When the Yin Chi and the Yang Chi meet, all body fluid will be exchanged and all the chi pathways between their bodies will be open.'

NINE DISASTERS

THE Chinese believe that there are nine situations under which people should not conceive. Called the Nine Disasters, these situations can lead to numerous problems, including miscarriage, stillbirth, a difficult pregnancy or labor, a physically or mentally handicapped child, or even a child with a negative temperament or perpetual bad luck.

MIDDLE OF THE DAY

Yes, when you make love is a matter of personal preference. However, from a procreative point of view, ancient Chinese healers believe that sex during midday—a time in China that is reserved for physical labor—disrupts the even flow of chi needed to create a healthy fetus.

MIDNIGHT

Some Chinese healers believe that the flow of chi is slowest at midnight. Sluggish, slow-moving chi makes it difficult for the reproductive organs to create the sperm and eggs needed for conception.

SOLAR ECLIPSE

During a solar eclipse, the sun is partially or wholly obstructed from view. To have sex when the sun is not clearly visible can create a disorderly, uneven flow of chi within the body, which in turn inhibits conception.

THUNDERSTORM

Any type of severe weather affects the earth's chi. Making love during these times can stop the smooth flow of bodily chi, causing it to stagnate in one of the internal organs. When this occurs, fertility is diminished.

LUNAR ECLIPSE

A lunar eclipse blocks the moon from our sight. To have sex when the moon is not clearly visible can create a chaotic, uneven flow of chi within the body, which decreases fertility.

BEGINNING OF CHINESE WINTER

In ancient China, conceiving at the beginning of winter meant spending the important first and second trimesters of pregnancy during China's most food-scarce seasons, winter and spring. For reasons of sustenance, the Chinese considered late spring to be the ideal time to conceive. This would allow a woman to spend the first and second trimesters during the summer and fall, when most of China's plant crops were harvested.

AT THE BEGINNING OF THE MONTH

The Chinese month is based on a lunar calendar, beginning with a new moon. The location of the moon affects the Earth and humans by its gravity and magnetic forces. Humans release different kinds of chi at different phases of the moon, which can affect the fetus. There has been no research about this conclusion, but Chinese believe that the beginning of the month should be avoided.

MAKING A HEALTHY BABY

The Chinese believe that certain sexual positions can increase or decrease a woman's chances of conceiving a child. Generally, positions that allow semen to stay in the body after intercourse are considered good for fertility, while those positions that allow semen to escape easily are considered bad for fertility. Couples hoping to conceive are told by Chinese healers to avoid positions where the woman is sitting, standing, or on top of the man. Instead, they should focus on positions where the woman is on her back with hips and legs raised. After intercourse, she is encouraged to remain in this position for an hour or more.

The Chinese believe that this pose forces semen to pool near the cervix, where it can better find and fertilize available eggs.

When having procreative sex, a man should thrust carefully to avoid spilling any liquid. After climaxing, he should wait a minute before withdrawing; in fact, the Chinese believe that after orgasm he should continue thrusting to further push his semen into the uterus. If he can make his partner climax, even better, as the female orgasm is believed to force semen high into the uterus. Lastly, a man should withdraw his penis slowly to avoid spilling any liquid.

WHILE DRUNK OR UNDER THE INFLUENCE OF DRUGS

Alcohol and other intoxicants cause irregular chi within the body, which may make it difficult to conceive.

WITH A FULL STOMACH

After eating, blood rushes to the stomach and the body expends its chi on digestion, leaving less chi for other pursuits, such as making sperm or releasing eggs from the ovaries.

THE SITTING MONTH

Every culture has its own protocol for new mothers. Some of these customs—staying out of cold weather with the infant, for instance—translate effortlessly across cultures, while others remain popular only in the country of origin. A tradition of the latter type is called The Sitting Month, a Chinese ritual that requires a new mother to stay in bed for 30 days. During this time, she is not allowed to come in contact with water. The Chinese believe that water leaches heat from the body, which is why showering, bathing, even washing hands or face, are all prohibited. Should a woman ignore health risks and come in contact with water, tradition says she will develop swollen joints in her fingers. The swelling usually does not appear immediately, but develops decades later when a woman is in her 40s, 50s, 60s, or 70s. She may even experience spinal conditions or back aches in old age. If the water happens to be cold, the consequences are graver still: the new mother may develop more immediate symptoms, such as a fever and partial blindness.

ANCIENT WISDOM

Lady Su, author of the famed sex manual The Book of Lady Su, wrote that the best day for conceiving a child is three days after the end of menstruation. The best time of day is between one and two am. Other Chinese sex experts say that the hours between dinner and bedtime are the most fortuitous.

CHAPTER FOUR

BEFORE GETTING STARTED

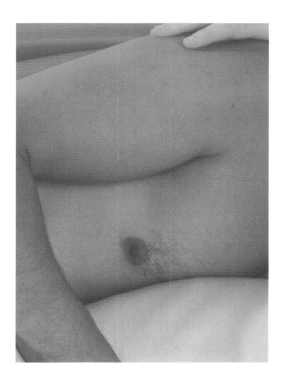

LIKE ANY OTHER PATH TO
ACHIEVING HEALTH, SEXUAL
HEALING HAS VARIOUS STEPS THAT
CAN HELP IN GETTING THERE.

CORRECT BREATHING

BREATHING is essential to all life. When we breathe we inhale oxygen, which is then transported to the body's cells and used for nourishment. When we exhale, we expel cellular waste as carbon dioxide. Proper breathing—full breaths taken from the diaphragm—ensures that all the body's cells will be well-nourished, including the blood cells, which rush

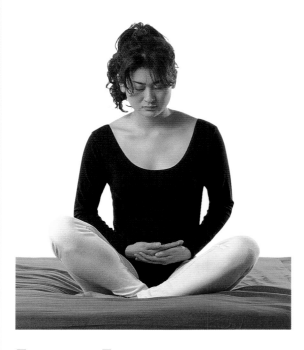

EMBRYO EATING

The Chinese have a saying, 'If you do not want a health problem, do not spit.' Accordingly, Chinese healers claim that the enzymes in saliva can bolster your immune system. Stories of people who have survived for months on nothing more than their own saliva are common in China. Embryo eating is done by keeping the mouth closed and continually swallowing whatever saliva develops.

to the genital tract during intimacy and engorge the area in preparation for sex. Furthermore, Chinese healers believe that proper breathing strengthens the kidney's chi—the kidney area being considered essential to proper sexual functioning.

In China, breathing is a fundamental part of good health. Proper inhaling and exhaling are among the first things a person learns when studying qi gong or tai chi. It is a key part of meditation. And it plays a role in sexual health.

As mentioned in the 'Reading List' on page 13,

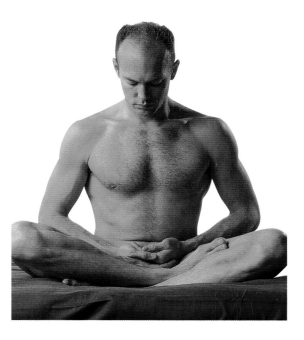

EMBRYO BREATHING

A meditative technique, embryo breathing is a form of deep breathing often taught in conjunction with qi gong, tai chi, and other Eastern movement arts. The procedure encourages the intake of oxygen through the nose, the mouth, and the skin. The latter may seem far-fetched to Westerners, but as the skin constantly absorbs oxygen through its pores, the practice isn't entirely implausible. It is difficult, however: it takes years of concentrated practice before one can properly perform embryo breathing.

during the reign of the Yellow Emperor lived a 100-year-old man named Peng Zu who looked half his age. When the Yellow Emperor learned of Peng Zu, he sent Lady Cai to learn the man's secrets. They turned out to be the following health-supportive sexual breathing methods

CALM, COOL, AND COLLECTED

A stress-free demeanor is essential for healthy lovemaking. When relaxed, we can focus our attention on our movements, our body's responses, and our partner. Unfortunately, stress is one of the most common health hazards we face today. It is nearly impossible to go through life without the irritations that make us tense. Furthermore, these annoyances can unexpectedly resurface in the bedroom. Fortunately, there is something you can do to minimize their power to aggravate you: deep breathing, which can be done anywhere and anytime you need to calm and center yourself. Here's how to do it:

1 Inhale deeply through your nose. Imagine your breath reaching the brain, filling the lung cavity, and traveling throughout the body.

2 Hold your breath for up to three seconds, then exhale slowly and completely through the mouth.

3 Continue as many times as needed. When in extreme disstress, take 20 to 50 deep breaths. Deep breathing pulls a person's attention away from a given stress and refocuses it on his or her breath. This type of breathing is not only comforting (thanks to its rhythmic quality), but also has been shown to lower rapid pulse rates and shallow respiration—two temporary symptoms of stress.

EXERCISES FOR MEN & WOMEN

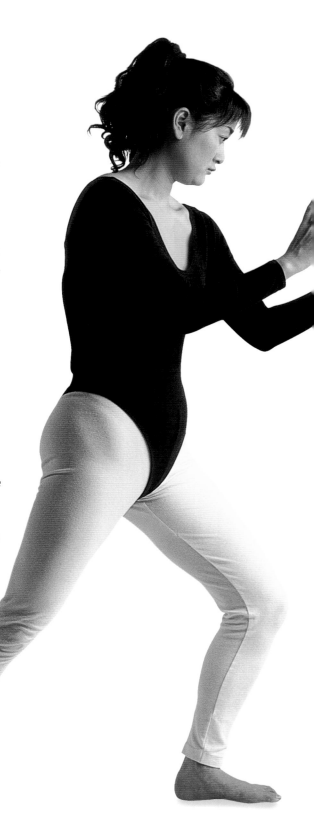

PHYSICAL fitness is not a romantic requirement. Plenty of people who have no stamina, strength, or flexibility have good sex. However, it is easier to have vigorous, long-lasting sex, and to enjoy a wide variety of sexual positions, when you are fit. In China, qi gong and tai chi are among the most popular national exercises. Both can boost your sex life (and your sexual health) by promoting strength, flexibility, and endurance.

TAI CHI

Tai chi, also known as tíai chi chíuan, is mentioned in the *Tao Te Ching*. The practice is derived from qi gong, yet, instead of solely promoting wellness, tai chi also encompasses aspects of Kung Fu. The discipline teaches a combination of tai chi forms that are performed in a slow, dance-like fashion. These ritual movements promote the flow of chi, increase self awareness, and strengthen and relax the body. Like qi gong, it is best to study tai chi with an experienced master to learn the proper stances.

Although tai chi consists of a series of positions performed in a continuous sequence, we offer the beginning pose to give you a sense of tai chi. The pose is called Salutation to the Buddha.

SALUTATION TO THE BUDDHA
Stand erect with hips tucked under and shoulders down. Turn your left foot out 45 degrees and sink down lightly on your left leg. Shift all your weight onto that leg and extend your right leg, flexing your foot. Cross your hands in front of your chest.

CONTROL YOURSELF

As the author of *The Book of Lady Su*, Lady Su was perhaps one of ancient China's best-known sex advisors. According to her, control was the foundation of a healthy sex life. 'Having sex is like riding a wild horse with a rotten rope. It is also like walking the edge of a cliff,' she wrote. 'If you loose control, everything is lost and there's no way one can maintain health and keep living a long life.'

QI GONG

Qi gong is comprised of a series of ways of brething that are performed in a continuous seqeunce. However, to give you an idea of what qi gong is like, we offer a sample exercise called Twisting the Waist.

Qi gong (pronounced chee-gong) is an ancient Chinese system of exercise created by early Taoists. It uses meditation, breath control, and movement exercises, much like yoga does, to balance the body's chi while strengthening the body's muscles. While qi gong consists of simple exercises, it is difficult to learn on one's own. Anyone interested is encouraged to meet once or twice weekly with a qi gong master to learn the proper posture and positions.

TWISTING THE WAIST

Stand with feet shoulder-width apart, and hold your stomach and hip muscles. Relax the shoulders and hold arms away from the side of the body at 45-degree angles. Rotate your torso to the left, allowing your left arm to swing behind your back and your right arm to swing in front of your waist. Repeat by rotating your torso to the right, allowing your right arm to swing behind your back and your left arm to swing in front of your waist.

FOODS OF LOVE

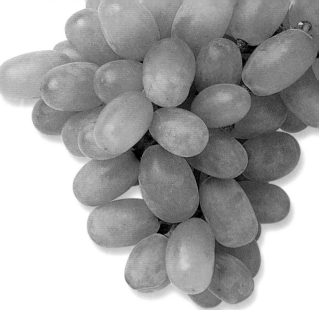

POMEGRANATES, asparagus, oysters, truffles, chocolate—in the West, these are considered aphrodisiacs, foods that make one feel romantic. Many of these edibles are erotic simply because of their shape—in the Bible book of Psalms, for instance, pomegranates are likened to a woman's breasts. Others, such as asparagus—a favorite seventeenth-century love food—are associated with romance because they are (or were) rare and saved for special occasions. Still others are chemical aphrodisiacs: oysters, for instance, contain zinc (as do many nuts and seeds), which help boost sperm count; truffles (the fungus, not the candy) boast a chemical that is nearly identical to a male sex hormone; chocolate contains a mild stimulant that helps heighten mood. China has its own aphrodisiacs. Litchis, grapes, walnuts, dates, and hawthorn fruit are commonly kept in the bedchamber and eaten before or during lovemaking. These foods are said to increase desire, promote endurance, and heighten physical feeling.

FOOD AND HEALING

In the earliest Chinese civilization, people ate whatever the earth offered with no thought given to what might be poisonous. Ancient books usually attribute the classification of edible plants to the mythical Shen Nong Shi (known as Holy Farmer Fellow or the God of Agriculture). Shen Nong is said to have personally tasted and tested a hundred herbs, and taught people how to forage for and grow nonpoisonous plants (it is likely that the clinical practices of ancient peoples were the real source of this medicinal knowledge). Around 3000 B.C., the Chinese began to categorize this information, defining a hundred plants that could be used as food, a hundred plants that could be used as medicine, and a hundred plants that could be used both as food and medicine. For example, hawthorn fruit is used in China as food and as a heart medicine, while Chinese dates are both a popular snack and a treatment for boosting red blood cell counts. The same categories are still being used today in Chinese medicine.

HERBS TO PUT YOU IN THE MOOD

Today, more and more people are turning to herbs to fight colds, boost immunity, heal wounds, and ward off heart attacks. They also use herbs to help increase sexual functioning. This may seem farfetched, but in China, herbs have been used for centuries to boost libido, strengthen erections, regulate sexual hormones, and more. Among herbal aphrodisiacs, these are some favorites:

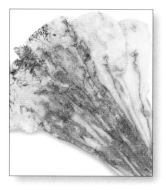

DONG QUAI

Many herbalists claim that dong quai has helped women conceive after unexplained infertility. The herb has been used historically by women in China (as well as Korea and Japan), as the main ingredient in a soup that is said to promote fertility. Unfortunately, no large-scale study has been done on the subject. Currently, the Western medical establishment views dong quai's fertility-boosting ability as anecdotal. Before using dong quai, talk to your doctor. The dosage is one 200-mg capsule three times a day. Because dong quai is a uterine stimulant, stop use immediately if you suspect you are pregnant. Dong quai is also used for female chi-flow problems such as painful periods, irregular periods, and heavy menstrual bleeding.

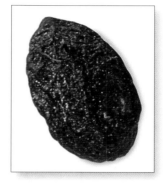

SAW PALMETTO

While not a Chinese herb, saw palmetto is the traditional Native American treatment for low libido, another term for low sex drive. However, the herb's effects are purely anecdotal; there have been no official studies examining the herb's influence on sexual desire. It is said that saw palmetto's tonic effects on the male and female reproductive system and the herb's hormonal action work together to create a desire for sex. Before trying saw palmetto, examine any possible underlying causes for low libido—such as a physical illness, anger, or low self-esteem. If there is no reasonable explanation for low libido, take one 160-mg capsule of saw palmetto two times daily. Continue as needed.

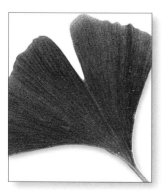

GINKGO

In Chinese medicine, ginkgo is regularly prescribed to treat impotence and enhance memory capacity. Indeed, several American studies of impotent men have found ginkgo effective in restoring blood flow to the penis, thereby helping individuals to achieve and maintain erections. The herb does this by dilating blood vessels, thus allowing blood to more easily reach the penis. With a doctor's permission, take one 40-mg capsule three times a day with food. Results tend to occur in six to eight weeks.

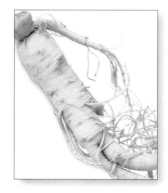

GINSENG

In Chinese medicine, ginseng has long been touted as a sexual rejuvenator and is regularly prescribed for both impotence and low libido. Several animal studies have found the herb to increase testosterone levels and sperm count, both of which can promote more sustained erections in impotent men. Ginseng has also been shown to increase sexual activity and mating behavior in rats. If there is no underlying medical or emotional reason for impotence or low libido, one 200-mg capsule of ginseng can be taken twice a day. Discontinue once erections or sexual appetite return.

PREPARING THE ROOM

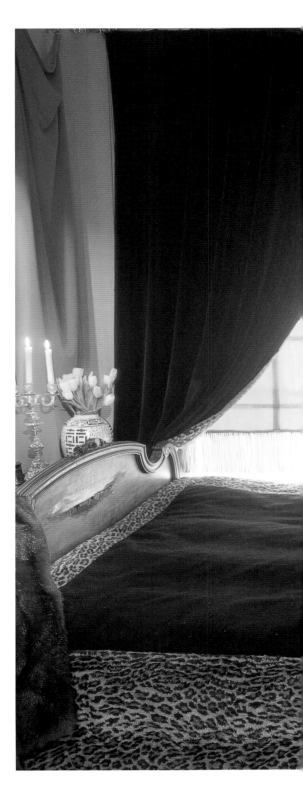

YOU are planning a romantic evening at home with your lover. If you are like most people, you dim the lights, set up an array of candles, light some incense, turn on the telephone answering machine, perhaps start a fire in the fireplace, and put on some soft music. These mood-enhancing moves work to soften the look of a room and make it feel inviting, relaxing, warm, and safe. After all, a welcoming environment is important to satisfying sex. It is hard to relax and enjoy lovemaking when the lights are too bright, the environment too loud, the room uncomfortably cold, or the air unpleasantly smelly.

Taoists give equal attention to preparing a room. In ancient times families lived crowded together in small spaces, making the most important preparation for lovemaking a privacy-providing curtain. Through the years, the curtained space has evolved into a curtain placed around the bed. This curtain creates the sensation of a smaller space, which the Chinese believe simulates the closed, safe feeling of an embrace. Curtains also are practical: They provide warmth, keep flying insects out, and provide an added measure of privacy. Dim light is another important element for lovemaking. According to Chinese healers, dim light helps humans feel centered, allowing them to focus their attention on their lover without being distracted.

The Chinese believe strongly in the power of smell, and regularly use perfumed pillows and sheets in the bedchamber. According to Taoist thought, fragrance helps heighten physical sensation. It also opens the body's chi paths to allow energy to flow quickly and smoothly.

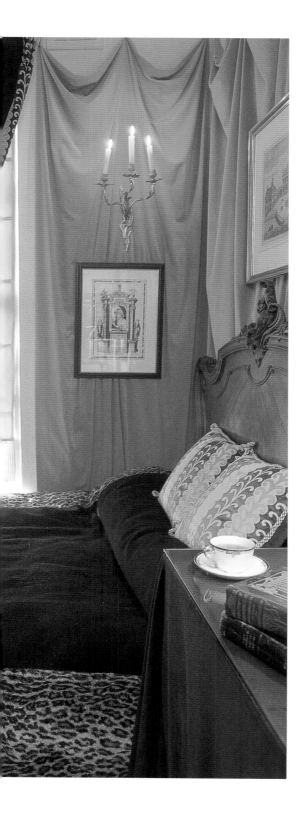

THE LOVE BATH

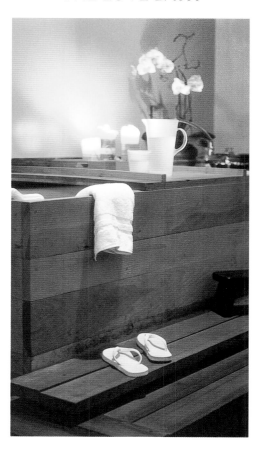

One of the most romantic things a man and woman can do together is bathe. A warm, scented bath can release stress, promote a feeling of calm, and enhance desire. It was common in early China for lovers to soak together in tubs steeped with flowers and herbs. In fact, the Tang dynasty empress, Yang, used to go—either alone or with the emperor—to a warm water spring in the Tang capital city of Xi An. She claimed that the waters improved the quality of her skin, her health, and her sexuality.

FOUR SIGNS OF A MAN

THE Chinese believe that as sexual excitement builds, the chi in a man's body causes the penis to go through four successive stages. Known as the Four Signs of a Man, they are as follows:

1 HE CHI (STRONG)

The penis loses its flaccidity and begins to grow firm when a man's chi moves from the kidney to the heart. It takes longer for the chi to go from one organ to the next—and thus more time for a penis to become firm—when a man is over-tired from stress, work, or physical exertion.

2 JI CHI (BIG)

The penis grows in size when the chi moves from the heart into the internal organs and then begins circulating through the body's muscles. When a man's penis does not expand in size, it means the chi has not yet reached the muscles. This situation is often the result of strong existing emotions or a poor immune system.

3 GU CHI (HARD)

Sometimes a penis grows strong and large, but not hard enough for intercourse. This situation occurs when the chi has not reached the body's bones. A weak immune system, an existing illness, or a negative emotional state may be to blame.

4 SHEN CHI (HOT)

When the penis is ready to use—literally—it will be strong, big, hard, and warm to the touch. This last state is reached when chi reaches the man's spirit. If the penis is not warm, it is often because the mind opposes the spirit. It should be noted that the fourth stage is an indication of sexual readiness—it is not a sign that a man should lose control and climax prematurely.

THE POWER OF TOUCH

Touch is a very important part of foreplay, helping to excite and stimulate a woman. To best do this, the Chinese developed a prescribed way of sexual touching. They believe that touching should begin with a woman's arms and neck, move to her legs and breasts, and end with her genitals.

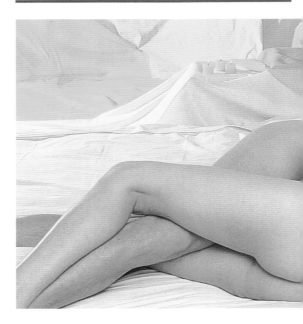

DOES SIZE MATTER?

In Western cultures there is a lot of talk about penis size, or lack thereof. According to this line of thought, the larger a penis is, the more desirable it must be. Fortunately, there is another way of looking at this. In China, a penis's size is always secondary to its power and energy. No matter how large the size, if there is no energy, a woman will not be satisfied.

NINE SIGNS OF A WOMAN

CHI has a great deal to do with sexual excitement. As chi progresses through the body, men and women advance through a series of sexual states. While men are thought to go through four such stages, the Chinese believe that most women pass through the following nine:

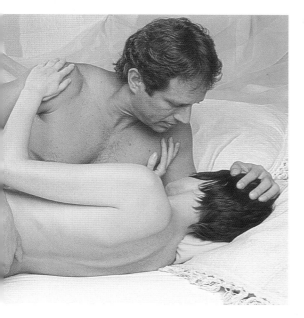

ROU (FLESH)

The Chinese believe that when a woman reaches out to a man and begins touching him, it is a sign that her chi is flowing freely over her skin.

FEI (LUNG)

In the Chinese medical system, the lung is the organ in charge of breath and swallowing. Therefore, when her chi reaches her lungs, a woman begins breathing harder. She also swallows her saliva.

GAN (LIVER)

When a woman's chi travels through her liver, she engages in full body contact with her partner, nuzzling him and pressing herself firmly against him.

PI (SPLEEN)

From a woman's skin, her chi flows to her spleen, and she tightly embraces her partner.

GU (BONE)

A woman presses herself tightly to a man and kisses him harder when her chi reaches her bones.

JIN (TENDON)

The tendon is considered one of the most powerful internal energy sources. When her chi reaches her tendons, a woman becomes more aggressive and may use her feet to hold onto a man.

XIN (HEART)

The heart is the organ responsible for emotion. When a woman's chi reaches her heart, she may sigh, her tongue becomes moist and she feels like kissing a man—either in specific spots, like his fingers, or all over.

XUE (BLOOD)

A woman touches her partner's penis when her chi moves to her blood stream. At this point, blood circulation increases, giving a rosy cast to her skin.

SHEN (KIDNEY)

The kidney is believed to control the front yin, which is the front part of the sex organs. Therefore, when her chi reaches a woman's kidneys, the front of her vagina becomes moist. In Chinese medicine the kidney is known as the major organ of sexual desire. A balanced diet and a low-stress lifestyle are recommended to keep the flow of chi moving evenly through the kidney.

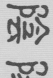

The
Art
Of The
Bed-
Chamber

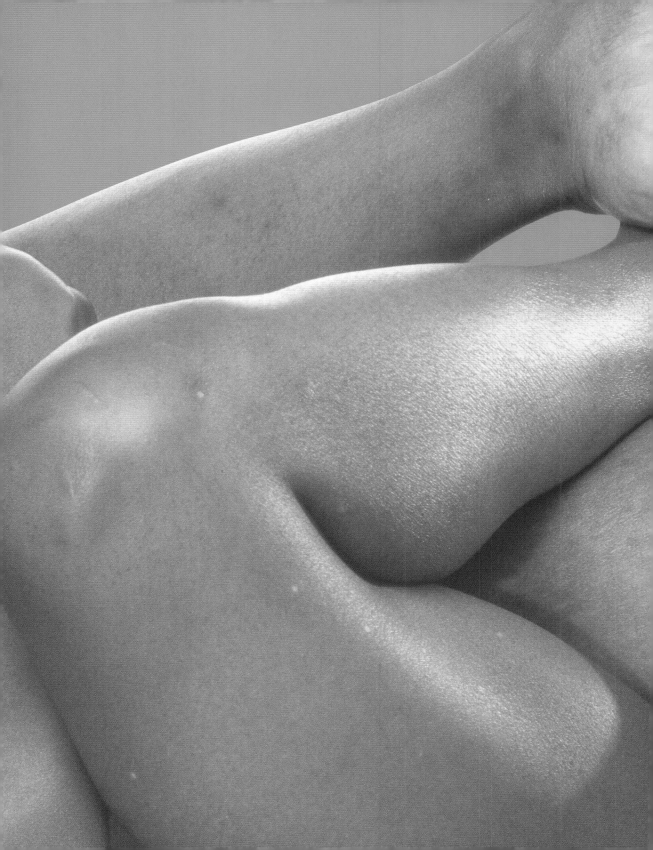

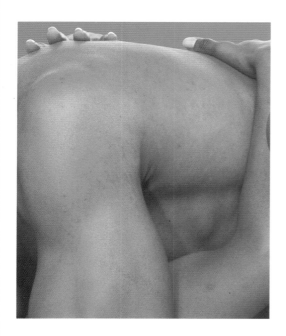

CHAPTER FIVE

ANCIENT SEX POSITIONS & BASIC POSITIONS FOR PLEASURE

SEX, ACCORDING TO ANCIENT
TAOISTS, IS A PLEASURABLE
ACTIVITY THAT CAN NOURISH
THE SPIRIT OF BOTH PARTNERS.

POSITIONS FOR PLEASURE

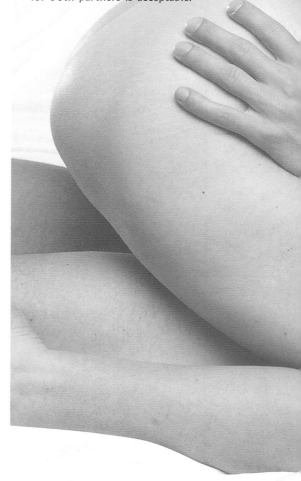

TAOISTS felt so strongly about this that they carefully designed a number of just-for-fun positions that ensured maximum sexual pleasure. The following poses, created by the Taoist philosopher Dong Xuan Zi 5000 years ago, help individuals better identify both their own and their partner's needs. The positions also offer an enjoyable way to deepen intimacy between lovers. Because these moves were designed as educational and recreational poses for healthy individuals, orgasm for both partners is acceptable.

CLOSE EMBRACE

HOW-TO In the Close Embrace, the couple lies face-to-face, arms wrapped around each other, for at least 20 minutes. Close embrace is a position designed to bring partners closer together; there is no intercourse. The touch of each other's hair, the smell of each other's scent, the gazing upon each other's faces—these all bring about increased intimacy.

ABOUT THE POSITION The Chinese believe that embrace is the first step toward emotional closeness and mental intimacy. Close embrace is especially important for new couples, but is also helpful for partners who have drifted apart and couples experiencing emotional sadness or stress.

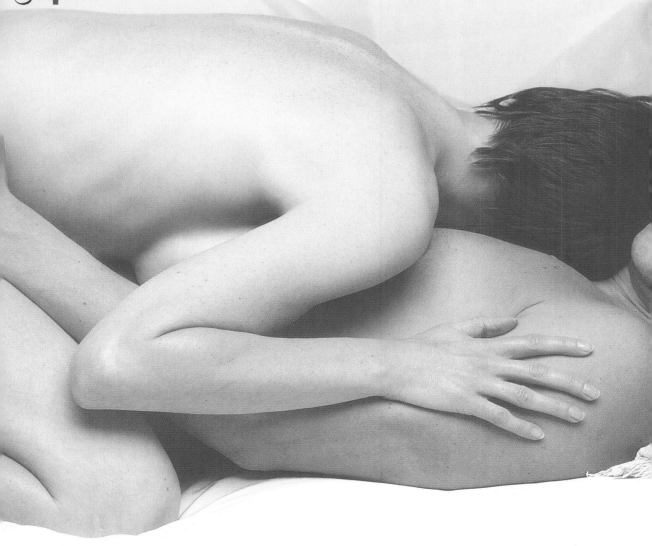

HOLD HANDS

HOW-TO In China the hand is considered a very sensitive and sensual part of the body. The sense of touch is most often associated with the hands, which are rich in nerve endings. The Chinese say that the touch of two people's hands is the silent talk between two brains. In the Hold Hands position, partners lie down or sit in a comfortable position and simply hold hands for at least 20 minutes. There is no intercourse in Hold Hands.

ABOUT THE POSITION This position is also referred to as 'wrapping.' Once a couple has successfully tried Hold Hands, they can advance to wrapping their arms and legs around each other. This will increase the amount of contact between the two, helping to stimulate more sensitive points throughout the body.

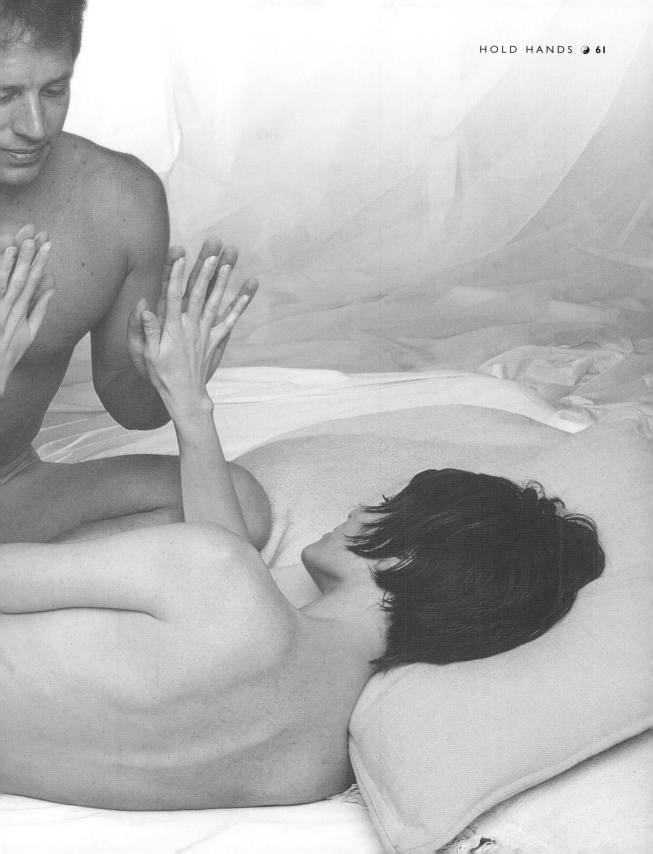

FISH FIN

HOW-TO Fish Fin involves what Westerners call 'heavy petting.' The objective of this exercise (which can be done with or without clothing and using any type of touch that is comfortable) is to build sexual excitement through body contact and physical stimulation without engaging in actual intercourse.

ABOUT THE POSITION When the vagina is excited, the Chinese believe it resembles the gasping gills of a fish that has been exposed to air.

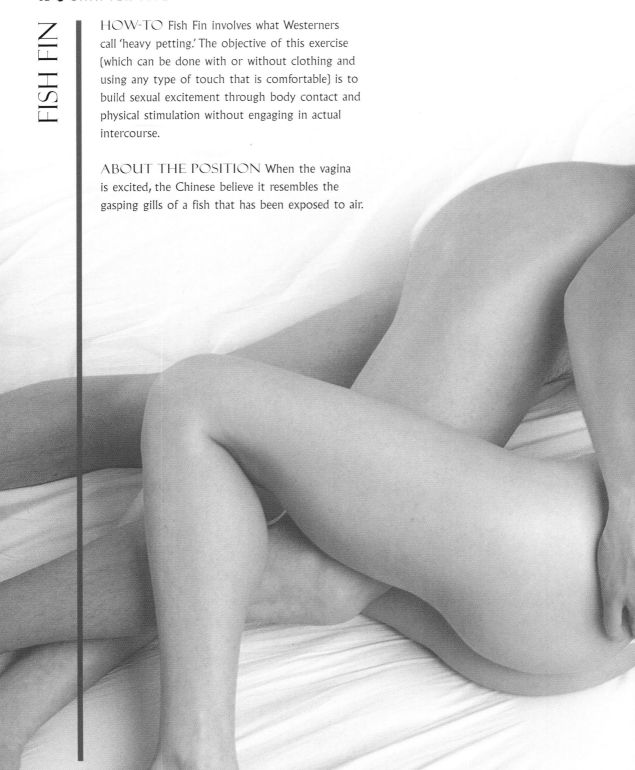

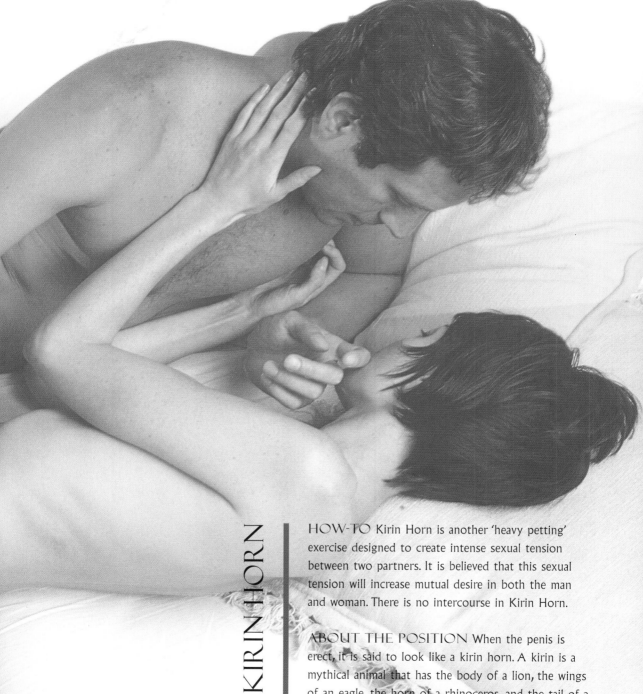

KIRIN HORN

HOW-TO Kirin Horn is another 'heavy petting' exercise designed to create intense sexual tension between two partners. It is believed that this sexual tension will increase mutual desire in both the man and woman. There is no intercourse in Kirin Horn.

ABOUT THE POSITION When the penis is erect, it is said to look like a kirin horn. A kirin is a mythical animal that has the body of a lion, the wings of an eagle, the horn of a rhinoceros, and the tail of a phoenix. It is considered a heavenly guard and is often seen 'protecting' building entrances, much like gargoyles do in America and Europe.

SILK WORM

HOW-TO The woman lies on her back. The man faces the woman and kneels below her hips. She wraps her arms around her partner's neck and her legs around his waist. After inserting his penis, the man can rest his forearms on each side of the woman's head. His thrust should be leisurely and gentle with constant kissing.

ABOUT THE POSITION Because it is gentle, playful, and non-threatening, Silk Worm is an ideal position for new lovers. The name of this position derives from the way the partners are wrapped together, which resembles a silk worm's cocoon.

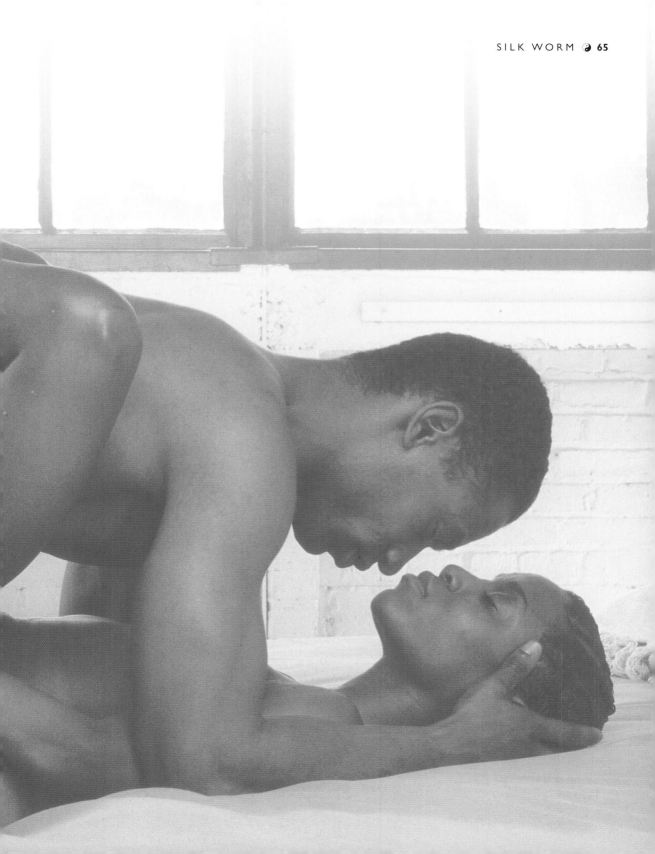

DRAGON TURN

HOW-TO The woman lies on her back with her legs bent at the knees and held against her chest. She holds her feet high, away from her body. The man faces the woman and kneels below her hips. Holding her tight, the man inserts his penis, experimenting with deep and shallow thrusts. Pressing and holding the woman tightly will make it easier for the man to control his movements, allowing his thrusts to touch different parts of the vagina.

ABOUT THE POSITION The Dragon Turn is so named because the Chinese believe it resembles the mythical creature, which has long limbs and a flexible body.

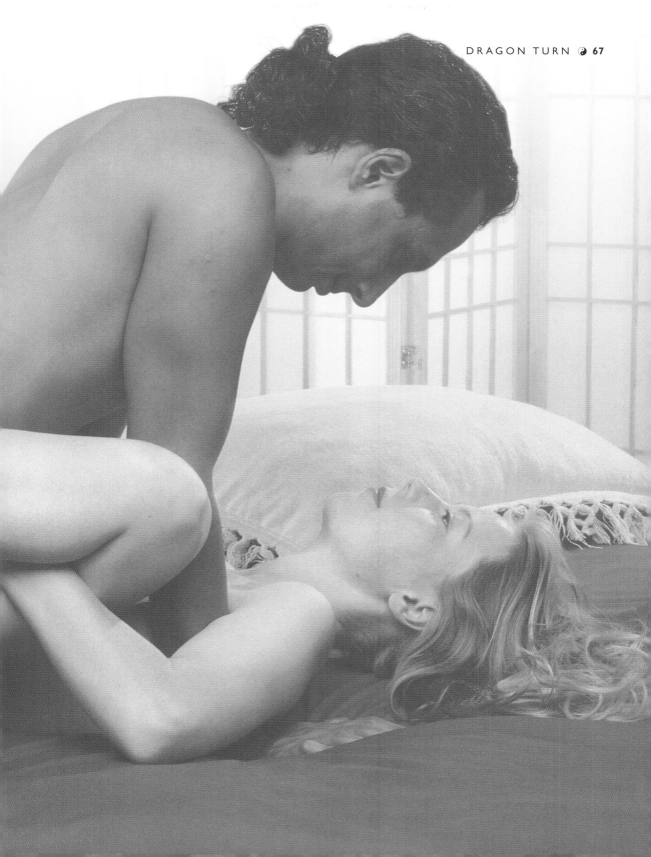

TWO FISH

HOW-TO The couple lies side by-side, facing each other. The woman wraps one leg around the man's hip. He inserts his penis, then holds onto her raised leg. Since the length of the man's penis and the depth of the woman's vagina affect each partner's sexual sensations, the man should experiment with both shallow and deep thrusts until finding a type of thrust that suits both individuals.

ABOUT THE POSITION This position is thought to resemble two flounder fish swimming side by side. It is an especially nice position for deepening intimacy between partners, as it allows the couple to look at each other and kiss during intercourse.

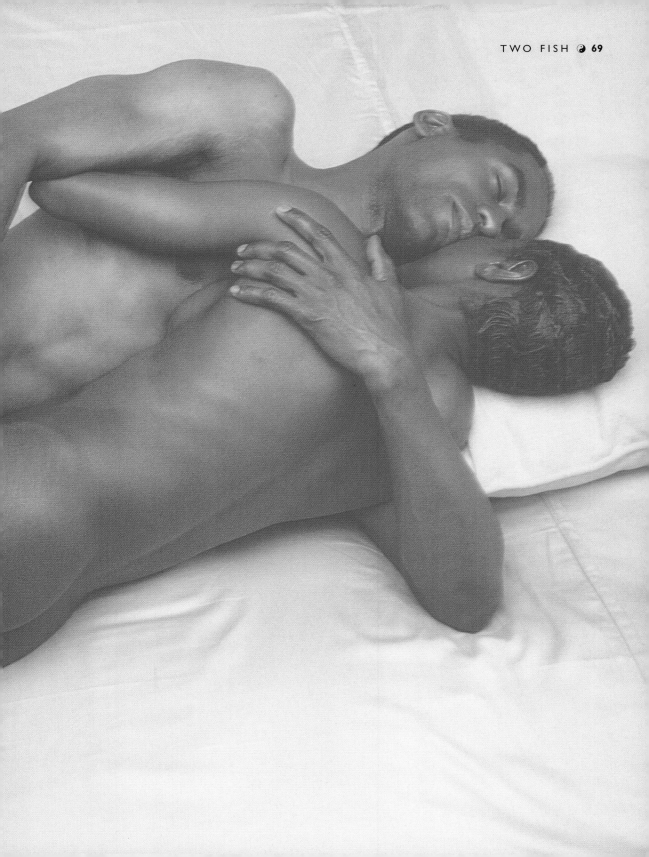

SWALLOW

HOW-TO The woman lies on her back with her legs straight and spread slightly. Facing his partner, the man lowers himself above her and positions his arms above her head, inserting his penis into her vagina. She holds his hips, helping him move. To help steady herself, the woman can brace her feet against a wall or the bed's headboard or grasp the top of her thighs; this may make it easier for women with weak legs to move their hips.

ABOUT THE POSITION The Swallow allows a man to touch his partner's clitoris with his penis. In this position, the woman's legs resemble a swallow's tail.

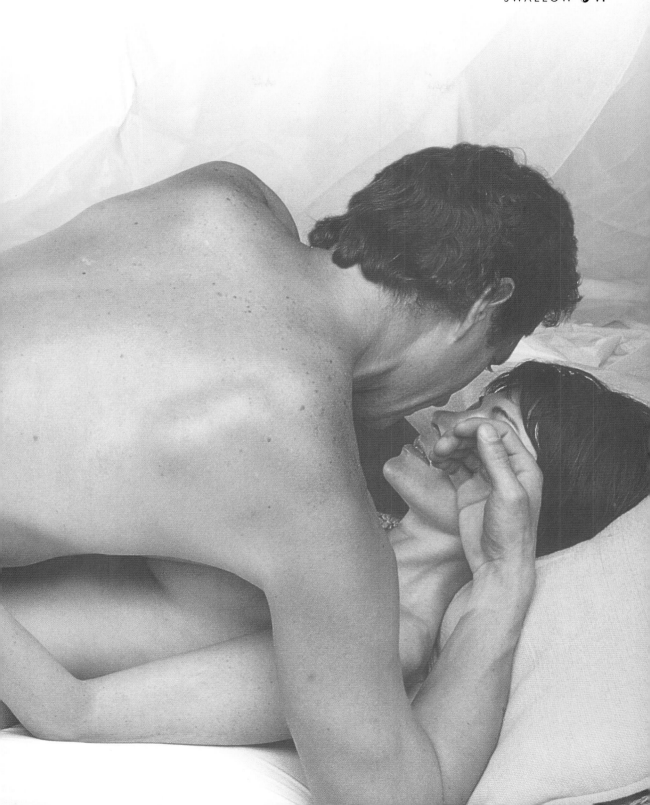

JADE JOINT

HOW-TO The woman lies on her side, bending her left leg at the knee and pulling it up to hip-level. She places her left hand behind her left knee. The man kneels below the woman's hips and inserts his penis.

ABOUT THE POSITION The Jade Joint allows the man's penis to touch the lower back side of a woman's vagina. In this position, the couple resembles a jade joint. Also called a jade cross, this is a Chinese art form where two jade pieces are carved and jointed together.

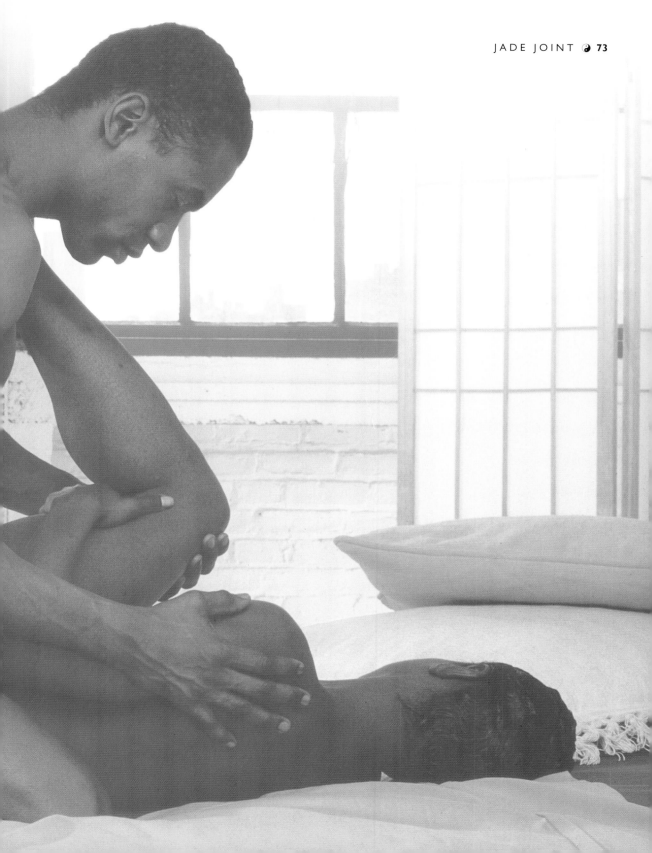

MANDARIN DUCK

HOW-TO The woman lies on her back, leaning to the right side, with her left leg bent and her right leg straight. The man faces his partner and sits below the woman's hips. He then stretches his left leg forward, under the woman's legs. He inserts his penis.

NOTE: A pillow placed under the woman's hips can make it easier for a man to enter her.

ABOUT THE POSITION Because they mate for life, mandarin ducks are considered the Chinese lovebirds. In China, the birds are used to symbolize marriage.

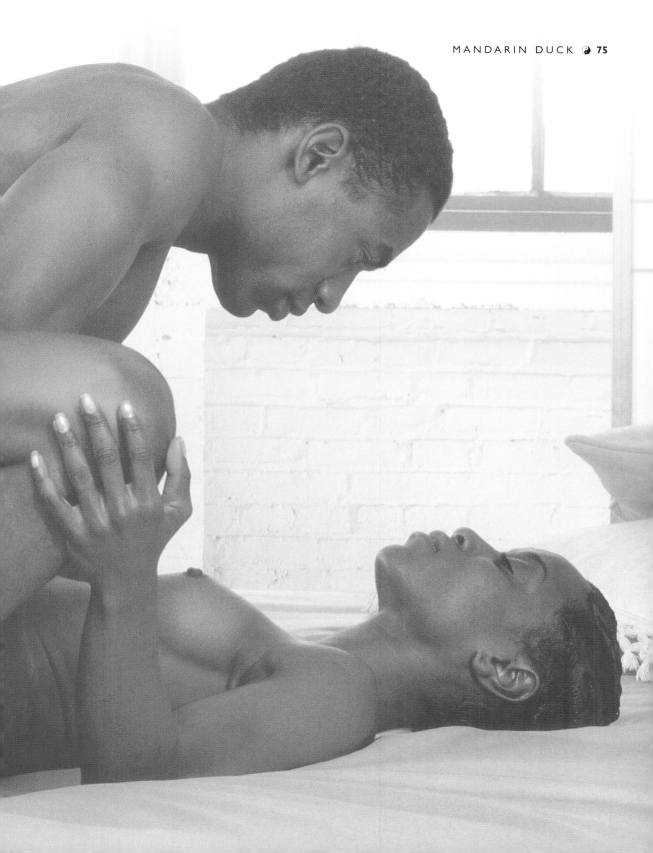

BUTTERFLY

HOW-TO The man lies on his back with his legs straight and apart. The woman faces the man and lowers herself into a sitting position on top of his hips. After inserting her partner's penis, she reaches behind her and grasps just below her partner's knees, which she uses to anchor herself. In this position the woman slowly rises and descends, using her legs to propel herself. If she needs assistance, the man can grasp the woman's hips and help move her up and down. NOTE: The woman should be careful to not hurt her partner's penis when she descends.

ABOUT THE POSITION With the woman moving on top of the man, the couple resembles a butterfly in flight.

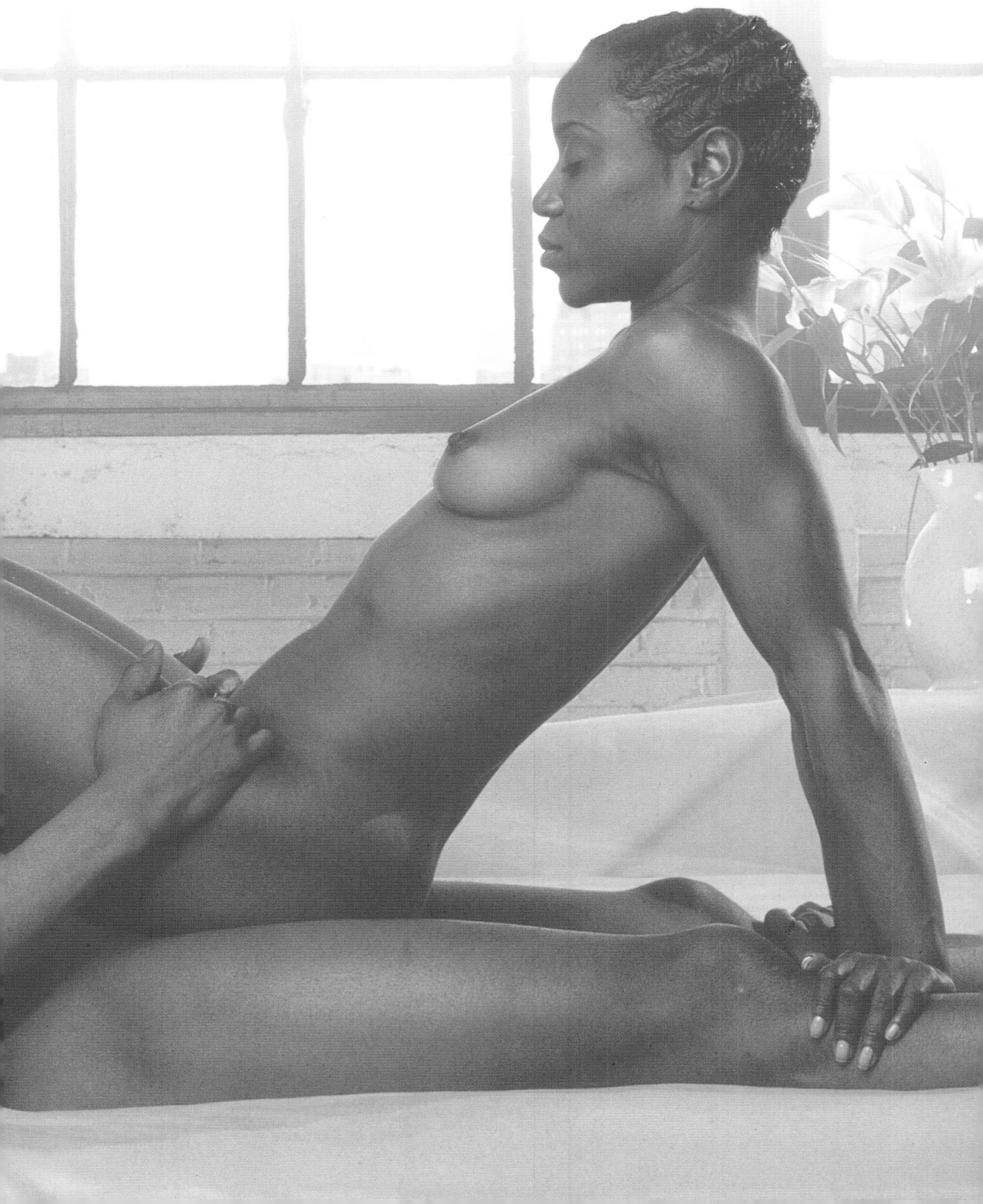

BIRDS FLY BACK ON BACK

HOW-TO The man lies on his back. The woman faces the man's feet and lowers herself into a sitting position on top of his hips. After inserting his penis, she bends forward slightly at the waist and lowers her head. She should hold her weight over her feet and raise and lower herself using her thigh muscles. If it helps, she can grasp her ankles or knees. If she gets tired, her partner can grasp her hips and help raise and lower her. The woman has to be very careful, because when she rises the penis can partially slip from the vagina, leaving it prone to injury when the woman moves downward.

ABOUT THE POSITION This position looks like two mating birds in flight.

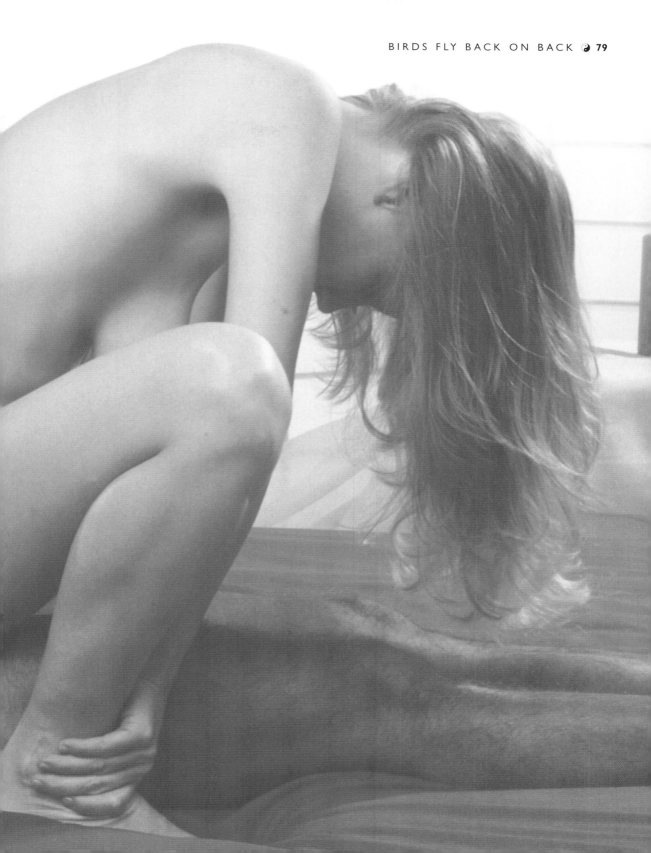

PINE TREE

HOW-TO The woman lies on her back, straightening her legs and holding them directly above her hips, then rests her legs on his shoulders. (Highly flexible women can try crossing their legs at the knees.) The man faces the woman and kneels below her hips. Reaching between the woman's legs, the man holds her waist. The woman reaches around her legs and holds her partner's waist. The man then inserts his penis. Unlike positions where the thrusting speed is left to the couple's discretion, in Pine Tree the thrusts should be hard and fast.

ABOUT THE POSITION Pine Tree provides a more intense physical experience than many positions. With the woman's legs raised, this position is thought to resemble a pine tree.

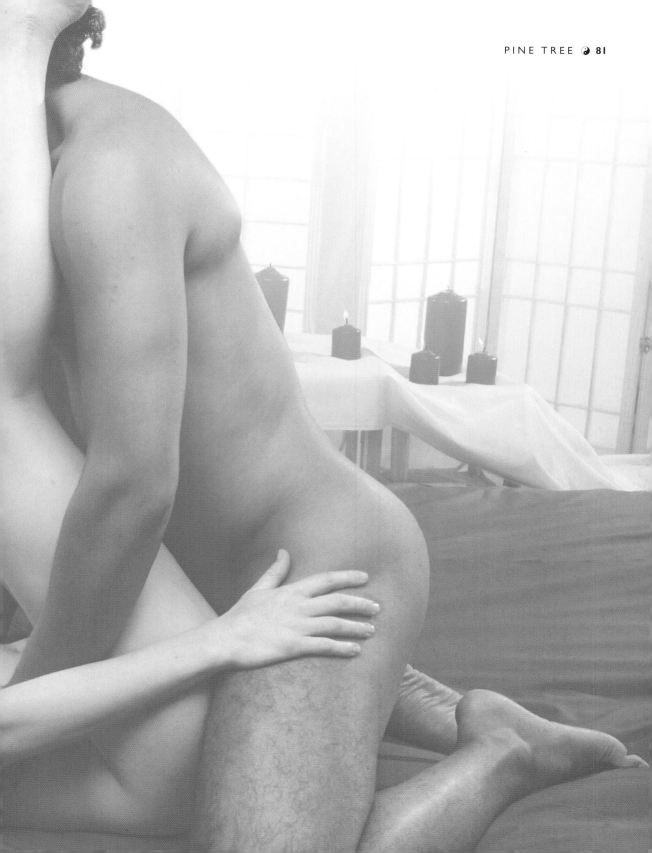

BAMBOO

HOW-TO The man and the woman stand
face to face. The man inserts his penis and
gently thrusts, embracing his partner if desired.
Because not all partners are similar in height,
the taller partner may need to bend his or her
legs and/or the shorter partner can stand on
an elevated surface. A man with a long penis
may also find it necessary to bend his legs
or ask his partner to stand on something.

ABOUT THE POSITION Because the
couple is standing, this position resembles two
bamboo stalks. This position allows the man's
penis to stimulate the front of his partner's vagina.

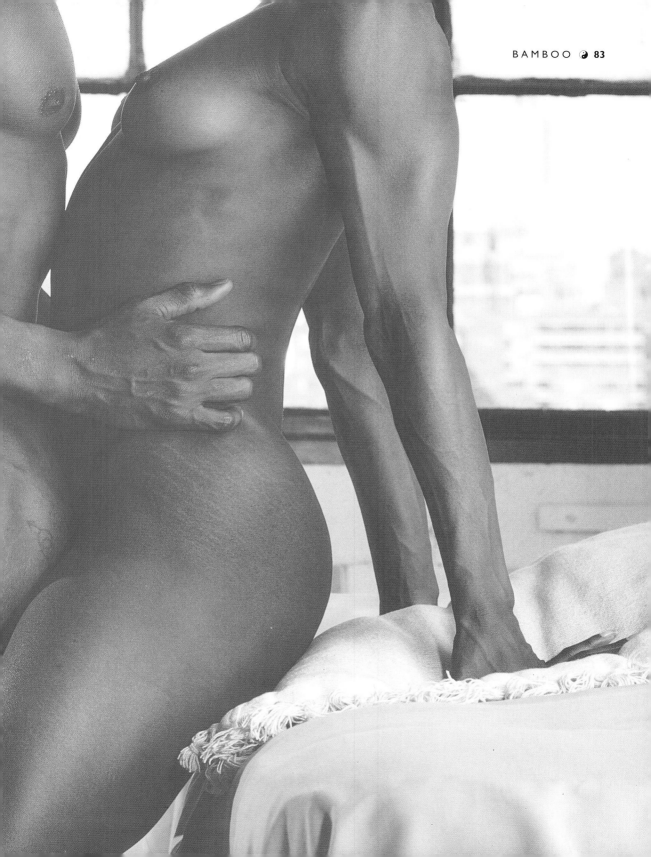

TWO FLYING BIRDS

HOW-TO The woman lies on her back. Facing the woman, the man lowers himself over his partner, supporting his weight with his hands and knees. The man inserts his penis and the woman wraps her legs around her partner's waist. If she likes, the woman can wrap her arms around the man's neck or shoulders or rest them above her head.

ABOUT THE POSITION Another version of this position has the woman on top, supporting herself with her knees and raising and lowering herself. The position is called Two Flying Birds because some believe it resembles just that.

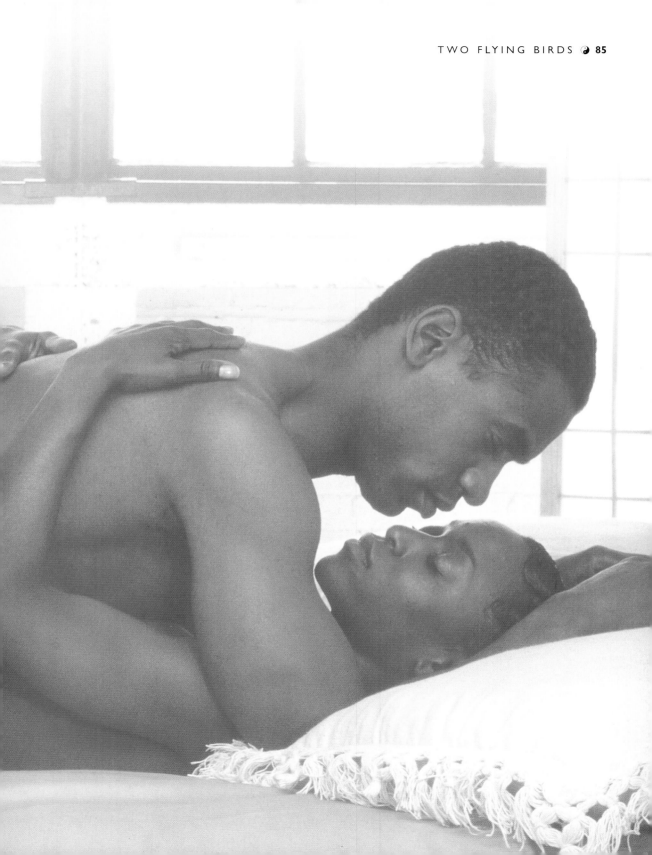

PHOENIX & CHICK

HOW-TO The woman sits or rests on the edge of the bed with her legs opened wide. Depending on a man's height and the height of the bed, the man stands or kneels in between his partner's legs, facing her. He inserts his penis and gently thrusts. If he likes, the man can hold on to his partner's shoulders or waist.

ABOUT THE POSITION The name of Phoenix & Chick derives not from the actual position, but from the participants. In ancient China, the position was recommended for a large woman and a small man—the heavy partner is the phoenix, the slight partner is the chick.

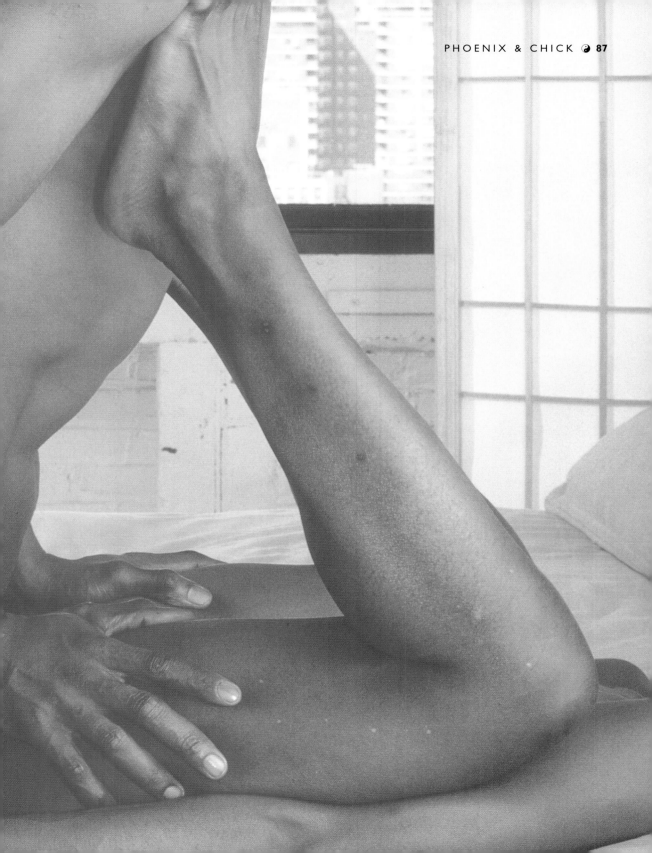

WILD HORSE JUMP

HOW-TO The woman lies on her back. The man faces the woman and kneels below her hips. Once the man is in place, the woman raises her legs and rests her ankles on his shoulders. The woman can hold her hand over the bedpost or brace her palm against the wall or headboard to hold her body steady. The man holds the woman's hips, inserts his penis and thrusts hard and fast.

NOTE: Some women experience slight soreness in their vagina the first time they perform this move.

ABOUT THE POSITION Wild Horse Jump brings the penis in contact with the back of the vagina. When the woman moves in this position, it almost appears as if she is bucking like a wild horse.

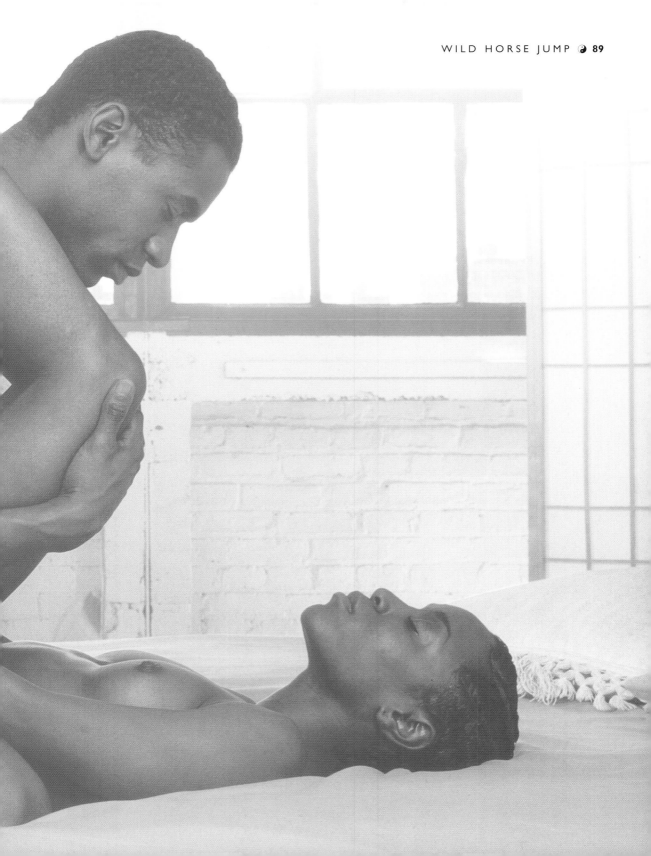

HORSE CROSS FEET

HOW-TO The woman lies on her back and bends her left leg at the knee. The man faces the woman and kneels below her hips. Once he is in place, he grasps her shoulder with his left hand. (Traditionally, the man may put his left hand beneath the woman's neck, but this must be done carefully.) He then clasps her left knee with his right hand, and inserts his penis. The man will thrust fast. If she likes, the woman can clasp her left knee and the man can place his right hand elsewhere. (If the woman finds it difficult to bend only one leg, bending both may make this position easier.)

ABOUT THE POSITION When a horse is running, its legs often appear to be crossing over each other. Because the woman has one leg bent, some think that the couple performing this position resembles a running horse.

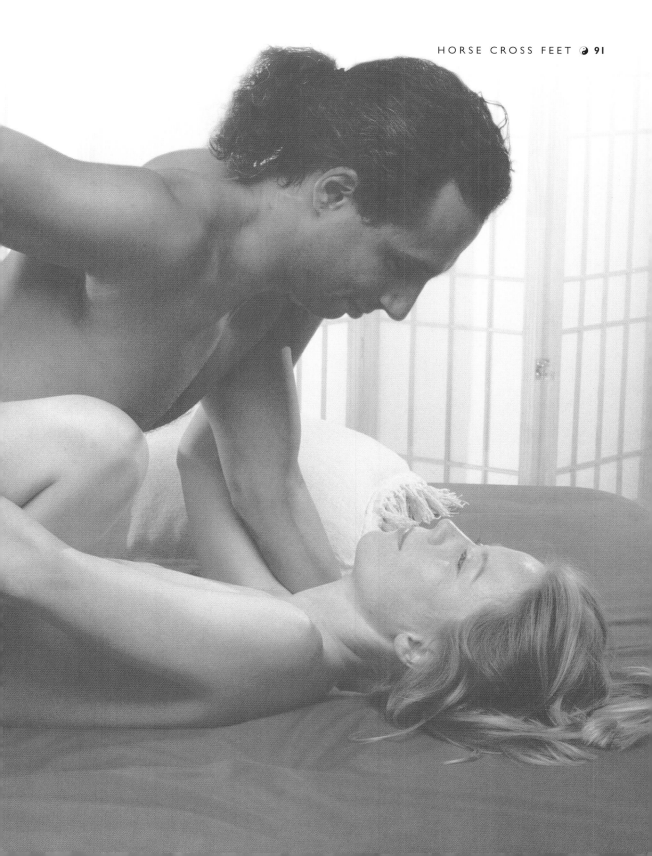

HORSE SHAKES FEET

HOW-TO The woman lies on her back. The man faces the woman and kneels below her hips. She places one leg over the man's shoulders while drawing the other leg toward her chest. If the woman is not flexible, she can use her hands and hold the leg near her chest. The man penetrates the woman and thrusts deeply. Some couples might find penetration easier when a pillow is placed under the woman's hips.

ABOUT THE POSITION Considered a playful position by the Chinese, Horse Shakes Feet allows the penis to penetrate the vagina deeply.

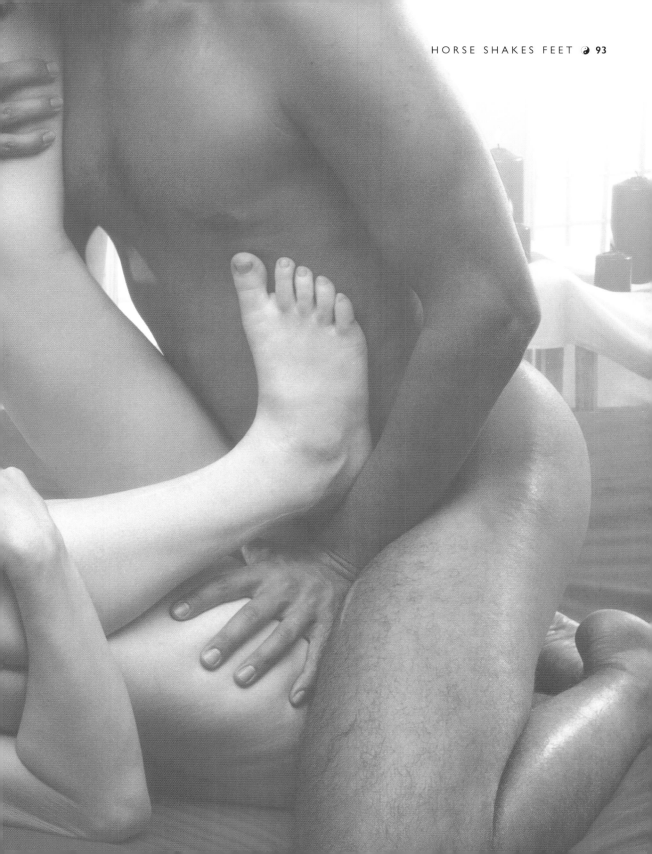

WHITE TIGER

HOW-TO The woman crouches forward with her legs bent at the knees and held shoulder-width apart, resting on her forearms. The man lies on top of her, using his hands to support his weight while inserting his penis. His thrusts should be a combination of fast and slow. In this position it is easy for the man to accidentally rest his weight on the woman, making her uncomfortable. Therefore, it is important that the man and woman remain in constant communication during White Tiger.

ABOUT THE POSITION White Tiger was so named because in this position the man moves like a male white tiger.

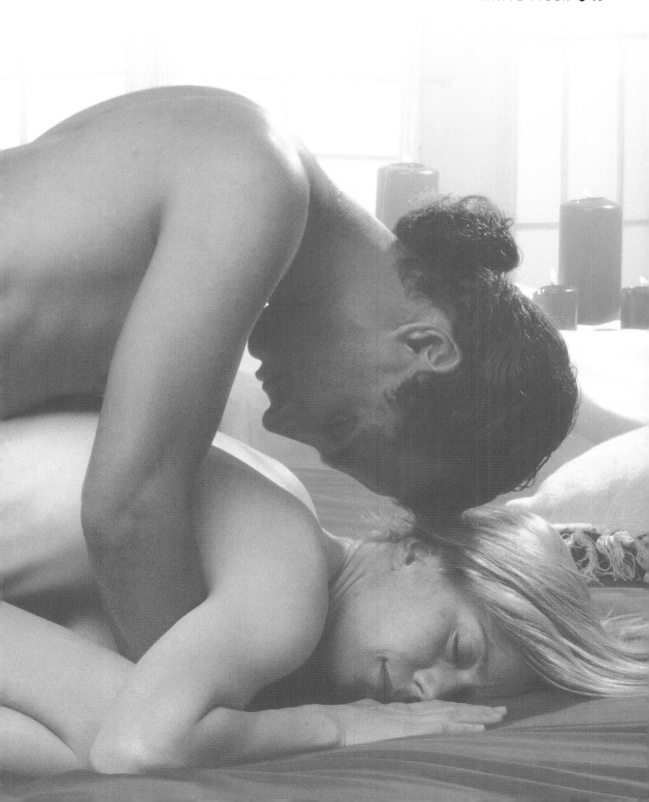

SEAGULL

HOW-TO The woman lies on her back with her feet at the edge of the bed, then raises her legs and bends them slightly at the knee. The man stands by the bed, holds the woman's thighs and inserts his penis. Because neither partner has to worry about supporting their body weight, both are free to move their hands and arms as desired. The man can thrust fast or slow, deep or shallow, depending on his and his partner's desires. NOTE: In ancient China, beds were quite high off the ground. If your bed is low to the ground, a table spread with a soft blanket or towel might be a better place to try this position.

ABOUT THE POSITION Some people find that in this position, the female partner looks like a flying seagull.

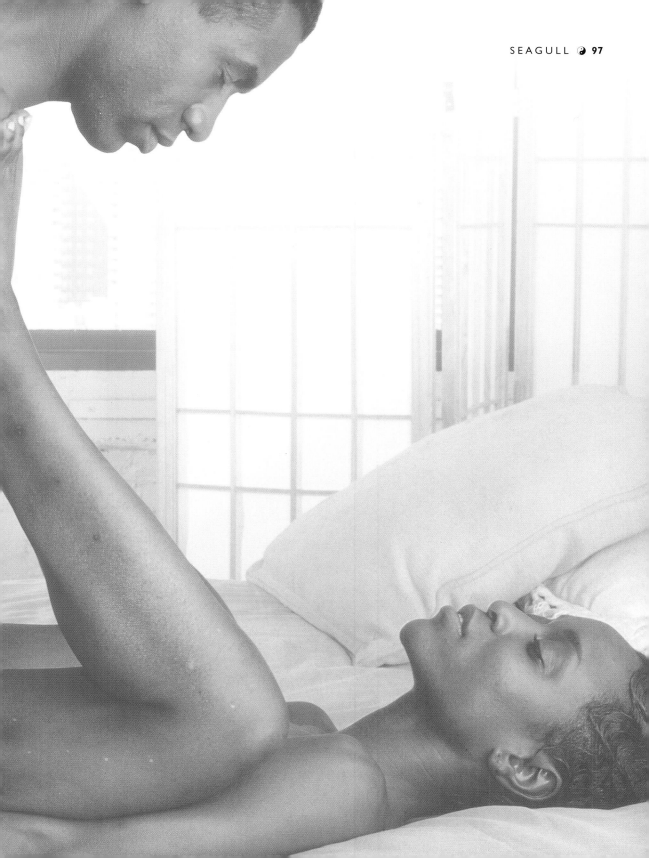

GOAT & A TREE

HOW-TO The man kneels down. With her back to her partner, the woman lowers herself onto the man's lap and onto the man's penis. When both partners are ready, the woman begins to move up and down. The man holds the woman's hips close and helps her movements. The woman should place her hands over her knee or her ankles. Goat & A Tree takes some practice to do comfortably. The first few times a woman tries this position, her thighs may become tired.

ABOUT THE POSITION This position can be especially exciting for a woman, who can watch both as she lowers herself onto her partner and during intercourse. Like all positions with the woman on top, the woman should control her movements in order to avoid hurting the man's penis. The position is named after a goat scratching itself on a fallen tree.

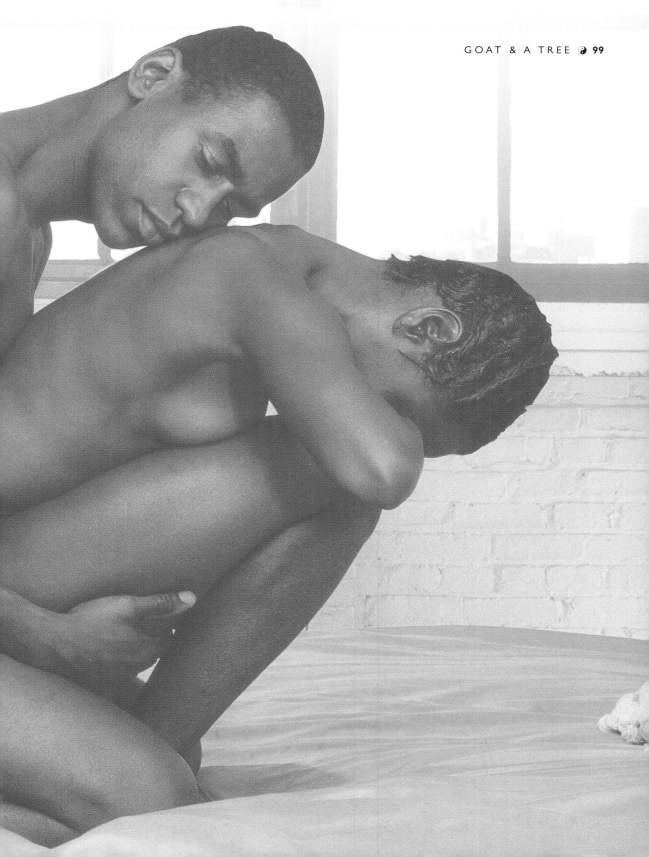

PHOENIX

HOW-TO The woman lies on her back and raises her legs, bending them at the knees. She holds her legs in place by grasping her feet with her hands. The man faces the woman and kneels below her hips. Once the man is in place, the man inserts his penis, supporting his body weight by placing his hands on either side of the woman's chest. He can thrust fast or slow, deep or shallow, according to the desires of his partner and himself. The woman is encouraged to move her legs in different directions to allow the penis to touch the inside of her vagina at different angles.

ABOUT THE POSITION The phoenix is a colorful bird with large wings and a long tail. The Chinese consider the phoenix to be a holy bird and a symbol of femininity. The Phoenix position allows a woman to move her legs, which resemble a phoenix's tail.

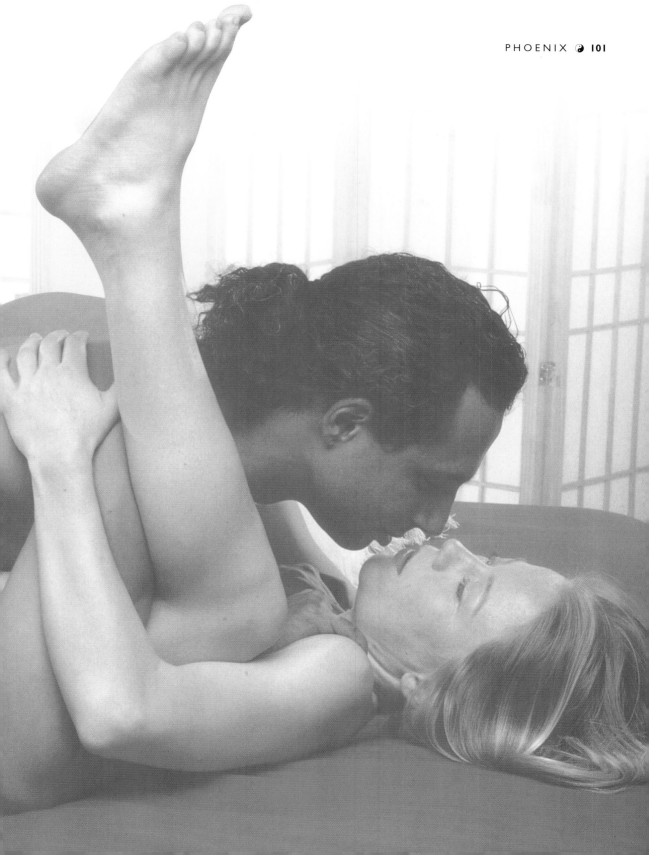

EAGLE OFF THE ROCK

HOW-TO The woman lies on her back and raises her legs, bending them at the knees. The man faces the woman and kneels below her hips, inserts his penis, bends forward over her, and tucks his arms into the crook made by her knees. He then gently grasps her waist and thrusts using a variety of deep and shallow thrusts. Since the woman's legs are wrapped over the man's elbow, the man has the more active role in this position. He may find it necessary to reposition his arms to support his weight.

ABOUT THE POSITION Eagle Off the Rock was so named because it resembles an eagle flying off a rock.

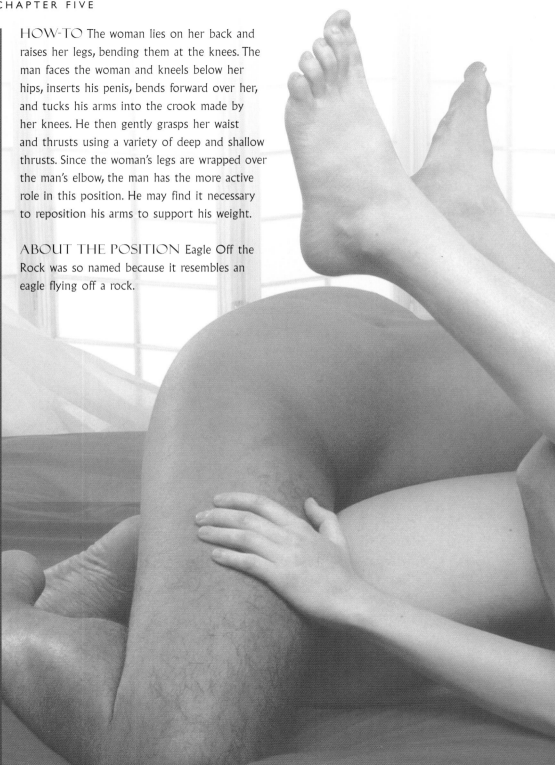

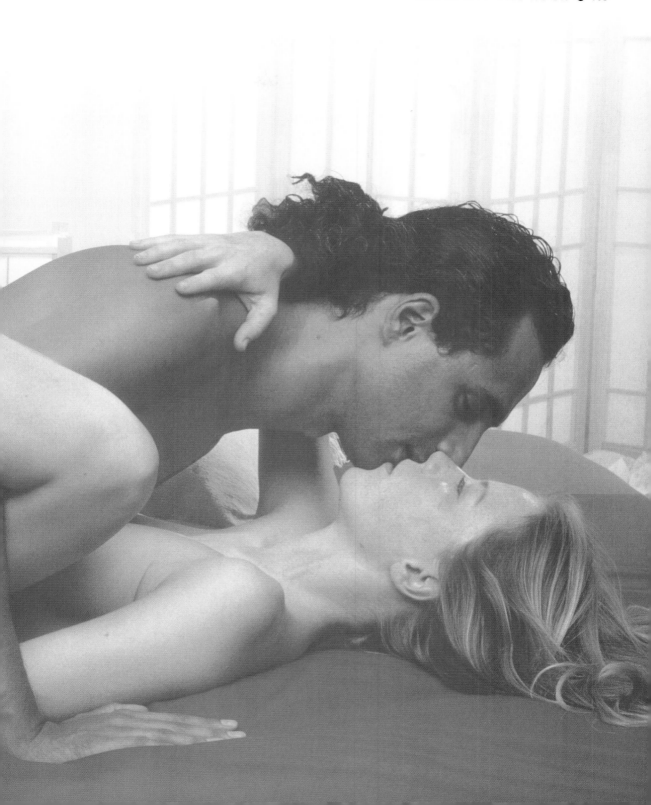

APE HOLDS THE TREE

HOW-TO The man sits with his legs stretched out in front of him, a little more than shoulder-width apart. The woman faces her partner, lowers herself onto his penis, and grasps his neck with both arms. In this position, it is the woman who moves. As she directs her hips left, right, up, and down, the man grasps her hips and helps her move.

ABOUT THE POSITION Different species of primates were often referred to collectively as 'apes' in ancient China. Ape Holds the Tree was named for the partners' resemblance to an ape holding a tree, a common practice among primates in the wild.

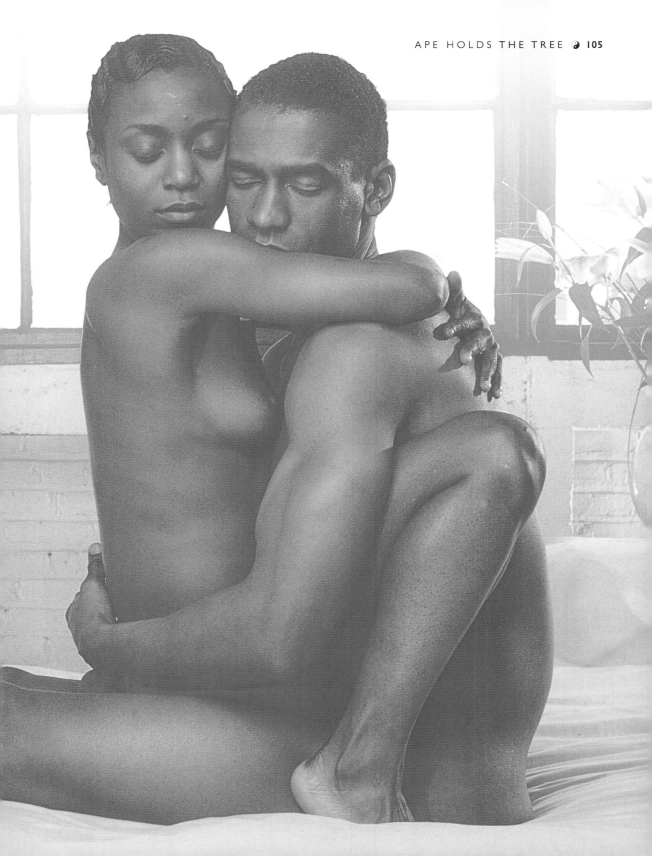

MOUSE & CAT

HOW-TO This position has several parts. To begin, the man lies on his back with legs opened shoulder-width apart. The woman lies on top and caresses the man, using the entire length of her body as well as her hands. After a while they switch positions and the woman lies on her stomach. The man lowers himself on top of her and lets his hands caress the length of her body. After stimulating her vagina with his hand, he penetrates her with his penis. The woman may need to raise her hips to allow her partner to better penetrate her. The couple may repeat changing their positions. The frequency of position changes depends on the couple.

ABOUT THE POSITION This pose is called Mouse & Cat because it simulates a cat playing with a mouse. The play between the couple helps stimulate sensitive spots while promoting sexual endurance.

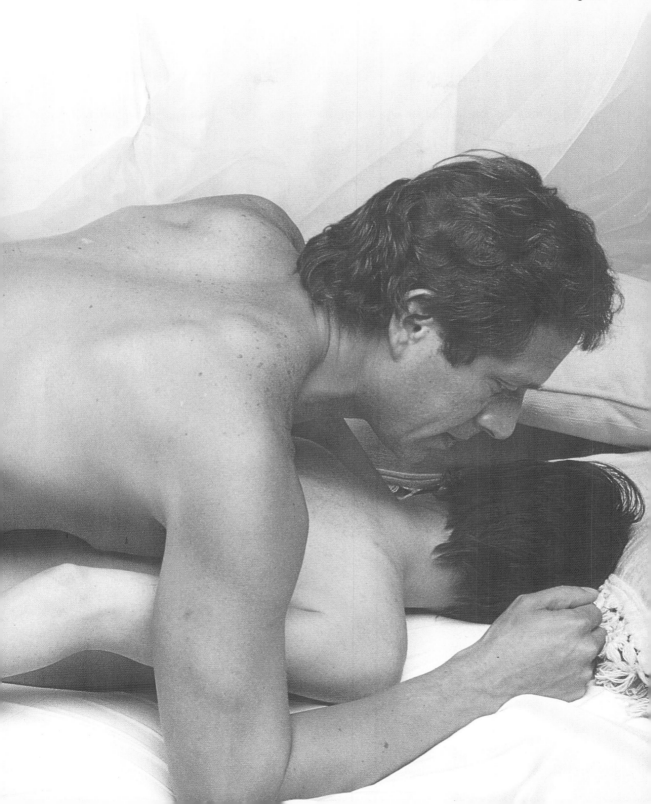

SPRING DONKEY

HOW-TO The woman kneels down on her hands and knees. The man positions himself at the woman's hips, grasps her hips, and inserts his penis. The man should experiment with shallow and deep thrusts, trying faster and slower speeds. This is a position used frequently in both the East and the West. It frees partners from having to support their body weight, while allowing the man to caress the woman's thighs, back, and breasts.

ABOUT THE POSITION In China, donkeys often mate in spring, which is how this position gets its name. This is a common position for most animals, referred to in other cultures as 'dog-style.'

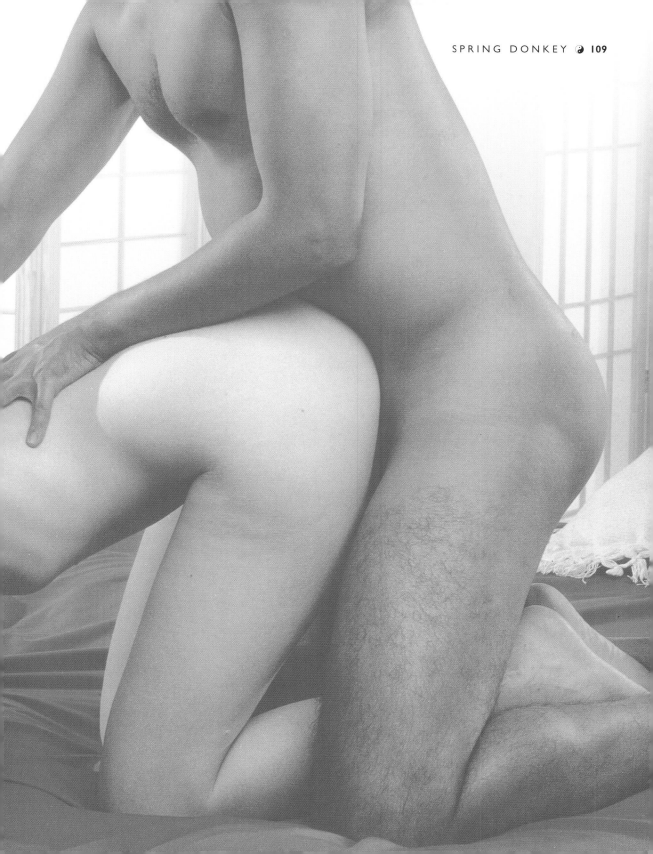

AUTUMN DOG

HOW-TO The woman bends at the waist, touching the ground with her hands. Next, she bends her knees, until she is able to place both forearms on the ground. Holding that position, she allows the man to back up against her. Facing in the opposite direction as his partner, the man bends at the waist, lowers his head, and carefully inserts his penis into his partner's vagina. Some couples find deep thrusts easier, while others prefer shallow thrusts. The position enables different types of thrusting.

NOTE: This difficult pose is a Taoist position in which size does matter: Autumn Dog is only possible when performed by a man with a long or curved penis.

ABOUT THE POSITION A female dog in heat will hold its backside high in the air. Often a male dog will mount either from above or the side, which is where Autumn Dog gets its name.

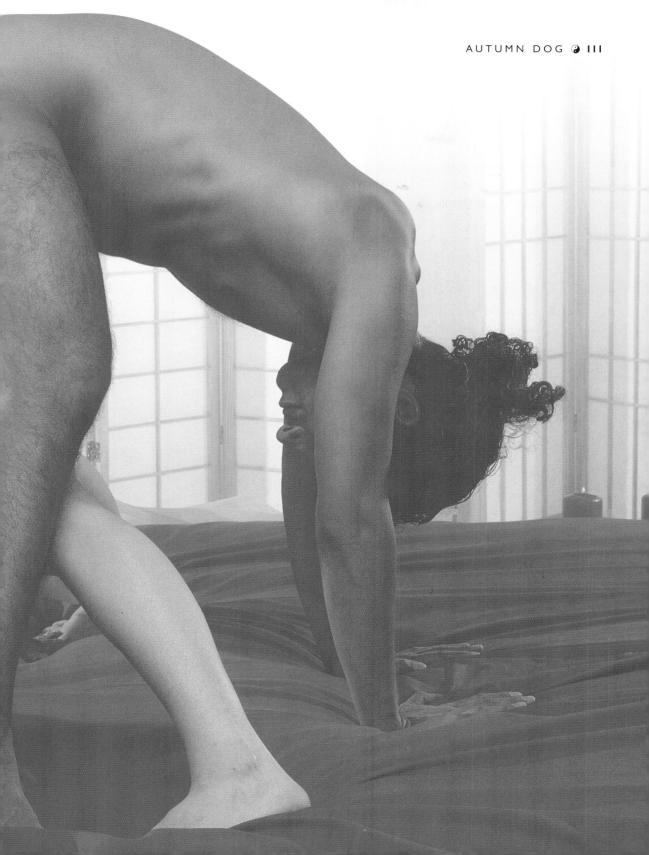

CICADA

HOW-TO The woman lies face down, raising her hips two or three inches off the bed. The man, also face down, lowers himself above her, supporting his body weight with his elbows and feet. He penetrates her and gently thrusts, careful to keep the movements shallow. Though the woman's movements are restricted, she still can move her hips to coordinate with the man's movements. Fifty-four was the ancient recommended number of thrusts required for orgasm. Everyone is different, however, and it may take fewer or more before both partners climax.

ABOUT THE POSITION This position is ideal for a woman with a deep vagina. A pillow under the woman's hips can assist her in maintaining the position and is especially helpful if her partner's penis is on the short side. The movement of both partners' legs resembles the beating wings of two mating cicadas.

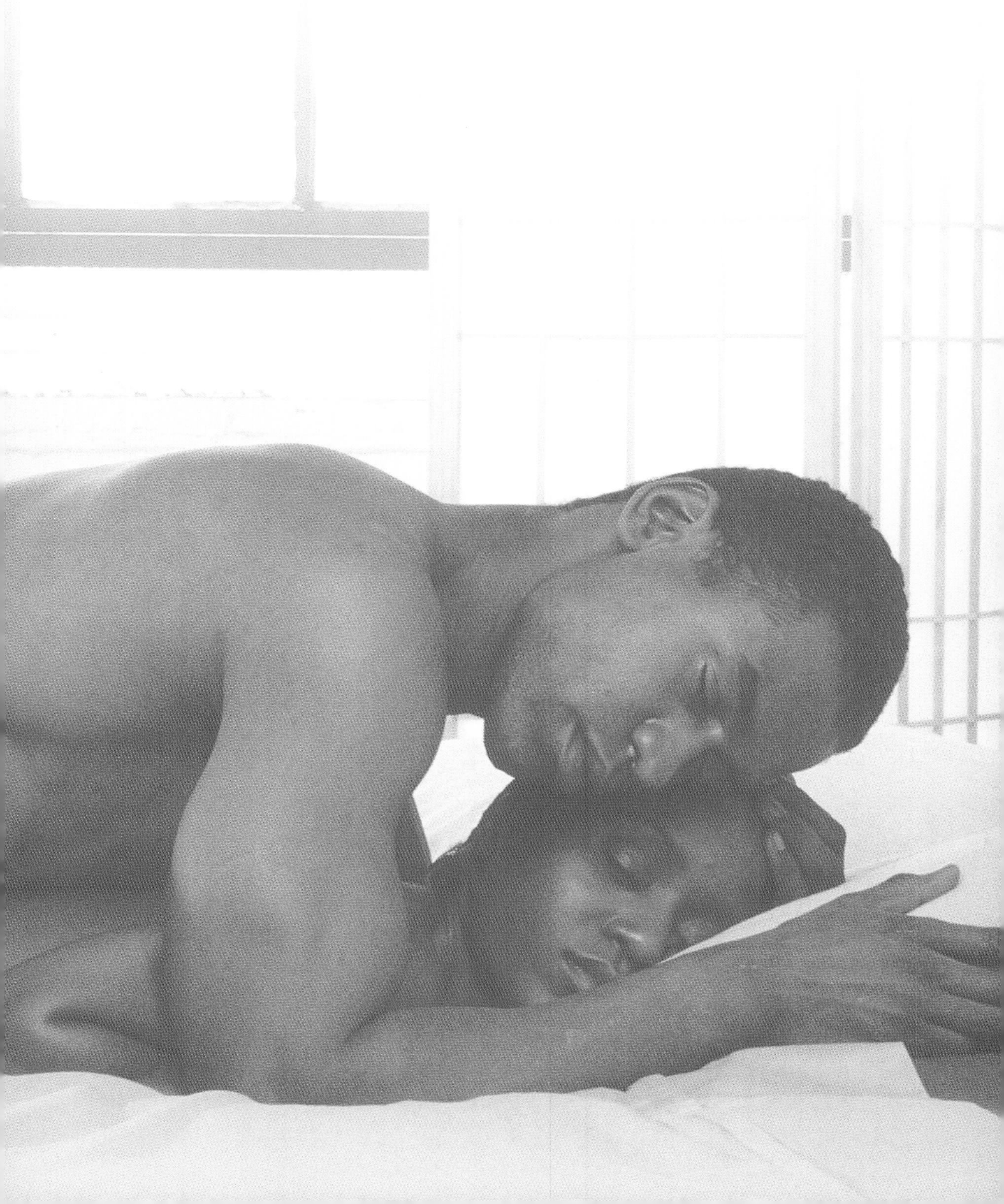

☯

CHAPTER SIX

MORE SEXUAL BASICS LADY XUAN'S WAYS

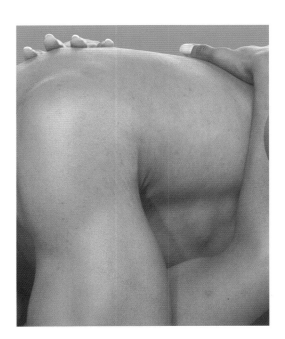

EXPERIMENTING WITH
DIFFERENT SEXUAL
POSITIONS IS BOTH SENSUAL
AND BENEFICIAL TO THE HEALTH.

EXPERIMENTAL POSITIONS

ACCORDING to Lady Xuan, a respected sex expert that lived during the time of the Yellow Emperor, a variety of positions increases interest in intercourse. Different positions also stimulate different areas of a woman's vagin, which is especially important, according to Lady Xuan, who believed that it took up to five years of experimentation for a woman to discover all facets of her vagina. To help a woman do just that—and to help couples add novelty to their lovemaking—she recommended various elementary positions. Because these positions were designed as educational and recreational poses for healthy individuals, orgasm for both partners is acceptable.

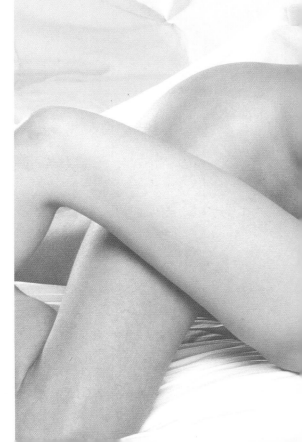

DRAGON

HOW-TO The woman lies on her back with her legs slightly spread. The man lies on top of her, places his legs between hers, and inserts his penis against the upper part of her labia. He then performs the eight shallow and two deep method. This method involves eight thrusts in which the penis is inserted only a third of the way into the vagina, directly followed by two thrusts in which the penis is totally immersed. Perform as many sets of 'eight shallow and two deep' as needed for orgasm.

ABOUT THE POSITION The Dragon puts an emphasis on touching. The yin and yang tradition proposes that the position increases a woman's sense of intimacy, allowing her to reach orgasm more quickly. This is a very common sexual position. Because the weight of a man's body is resting on his hands and knees, he looks like a dragon, hence the name Dragon.

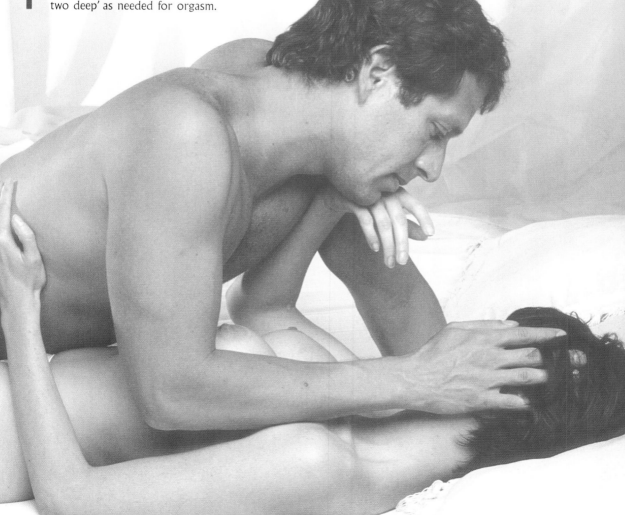

TIGER STEP

HOW-TO The woman begins in a kneeling position, raises her arms straight over her head, then bends forward toward the bed. Resting her arms, shoulders, neck, head, and chest on the bed, she lifts her hips high. The man positions himself behind her hips, kneels, and holds her waist with both hands. He inserts his penis as deeply as possible, thrusting quickly, approximately forty times. Just how many thrusts he performs depends on his and his partner's stamina and on how long it takes his partner to climax. When the woman reaches orgasm, the man can stop.

ABOUT THE POSITION In the Tiger Step, the man does not have to support his own body weight, leaving his hands free to caress his partner and to control the speed of his penetration. Since the couple performing this position looks like a tiger waiting for the hunt, it is called Tiger Step.

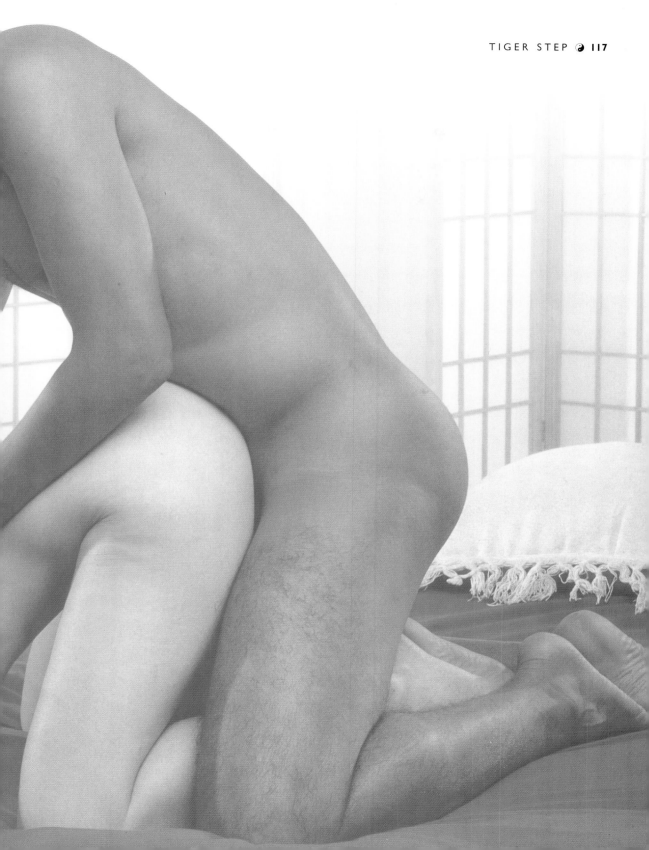

APE

HOW-TO The woman lies on her back, extends her legs, and holds them straight above her hips. The man faces the woman and kneels below her hips. She rests her legs over her partner's shoulders, then he places his hands on her buttocks and gently lifts her hips two or three inches before penetrating her. The thrusts should start shallow and gradually; as the woman's vagina becomes moister, thrusting can become deeper. Continue until both partners have climaxed.

ABOUT THE POSITION Many Chinese like this position: It shows the female labia, makes it easy for the man to penetrate the vagina, and allows a man to appreciate a woman's feet. Due to the vagina's accessible position, the fact that the man does not have to support his own weight, and that the male is not resting his weight above his partner, the Ape is an ideal sexual position for overweight men.

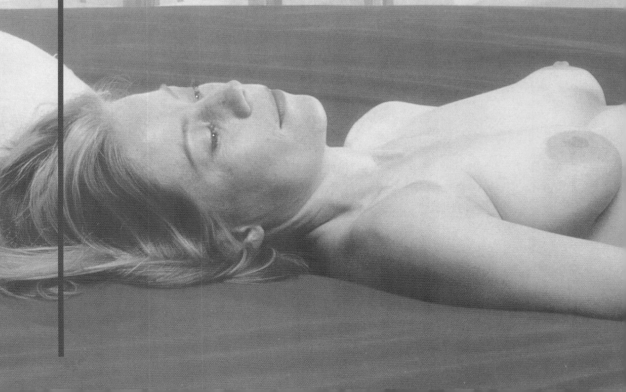

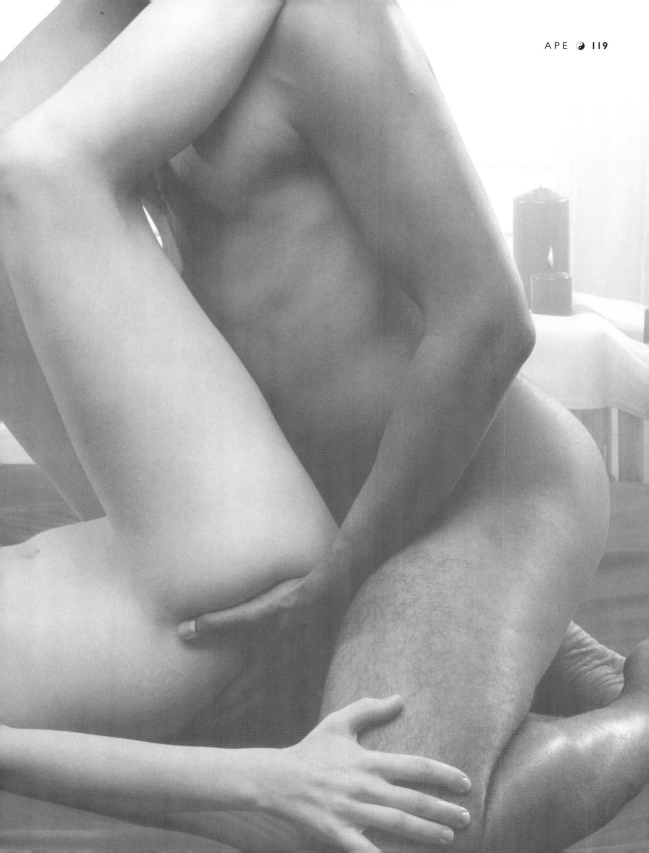

CICADA TO THE SIDE

HOW-TO Similar to the popular Cicada position found in 'Ancient Sex Basics' (page 112), Cicada to the Side is simply an alternative version. The woman lies on her left side with the man lying directly behind her, also on his left side. Embracing his partner's waist or chest, the man inserts his penis and thrusts gently, careful to keep the movements shallow.

ABOUT THE POSITION Cicada to the Side is ideal for a man who is feeling tired or who is too weak to support his weight. It is also a good position for a woman with a shallow vagina.

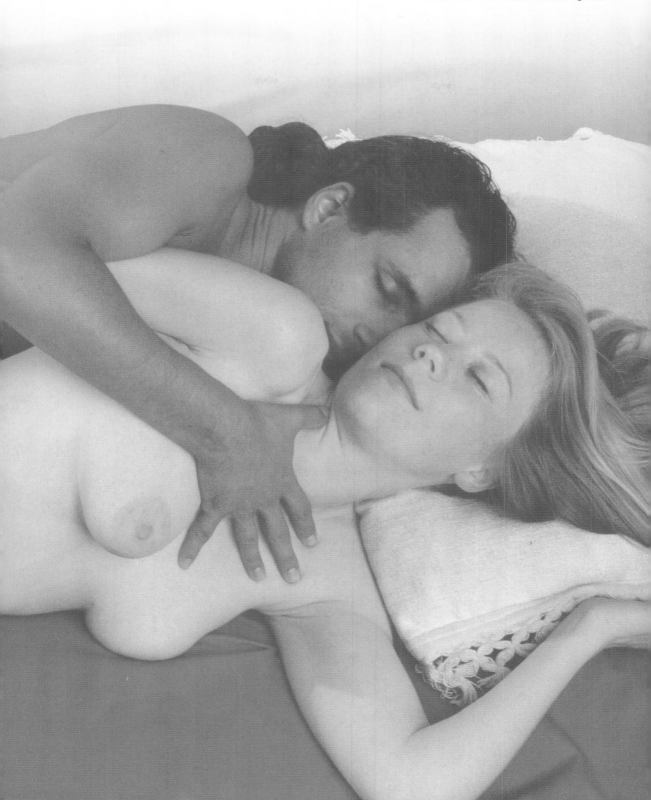

TURTLE MOVE

HOW-TO The woman lies on her back and bends her legs. The man kneels down below her hips and grabs her legs at or just above the knee. After he pushes his partner's legs forward, he penetrates her, continuing to hold her legs forward as he thrusts. His movements should be slow and deliberate and he should pull his penis almost entirely out before inserting it again.

ABOUT THE POSITION In the Turtle Move position a man holds his partner's body very tightly, allowing the woman to orgasm by moving her body in resistance to her partner. In this position the couple is believed to resemble a turtle swimming in the ocean.

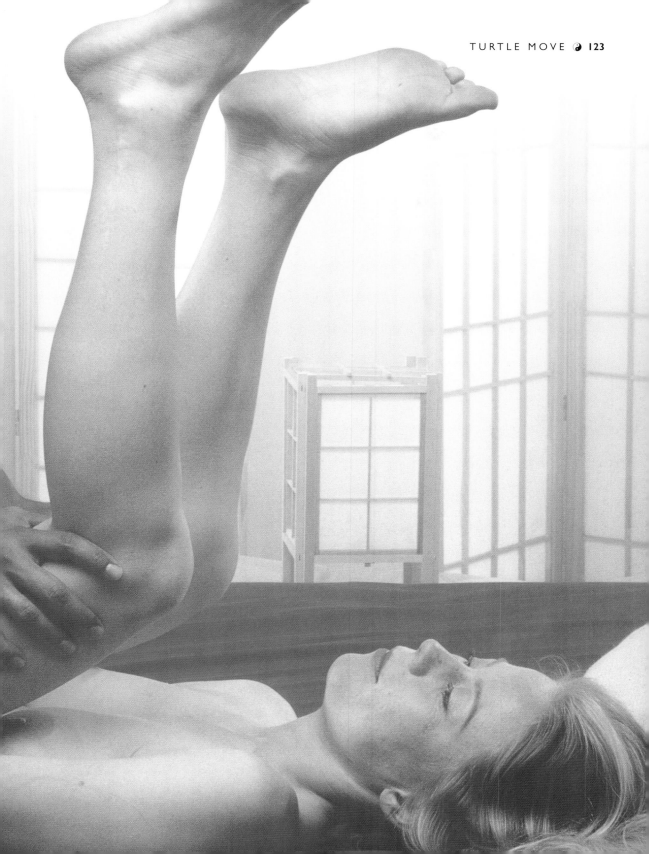

RABBIT GROOMING

HOW-TO The man lies on his back. The woman sits on top of him, facing his feet. The woman bends at the waist, lowers her head, and moves up and down, to the left and right. Her hands can grasp the man's knees, calves, or ankles. She will be able to move her hips with less exertion if she chooses to hold on to her partner's ankles. The man holds the woman's hips, and, after inserting his penis, helps to move it around. In this position, a woman must take care not to hurt the penis with a sudden move or an awkward thrust.

ABOUT THE POSITION A couple performing this position resembles a rabbit carefully grooming itself. Most women find Rabbit Grooming difficult on the first try since it requires a lot of strength from the waist to the legs. But because she is the partner in control, a woman may find this position enjoyable with practice.

LITERARY LOVEMAKING

The ancient novel *Jade Prayer Mat* portrays a very experienced woman whose favorite position is Rabbit Grooming. She prefers the pose because she can move fast or slow, left or right, depending on the sensations inside her vagina. She can also control the way her partner's penis touches her clitoris.

FISH

HOW-TO The man lies on his back with his legs straight. The woman sits on top of his hips, facing him. She moves a little bit forward and with her labia takes in the man's penis just slightly. The man does not move much. When she is ready, she inserts the penis and moves right and left, up and down (shown here).

ABOUT THE POSITION Fish is a favorite position of many men, who find delight in watching the movement of their partner's breasts. If he gently touches his partner's nipples, she may reach orgasm faster. The pose was given its name because the couple looks like a fish moving slowly in water.

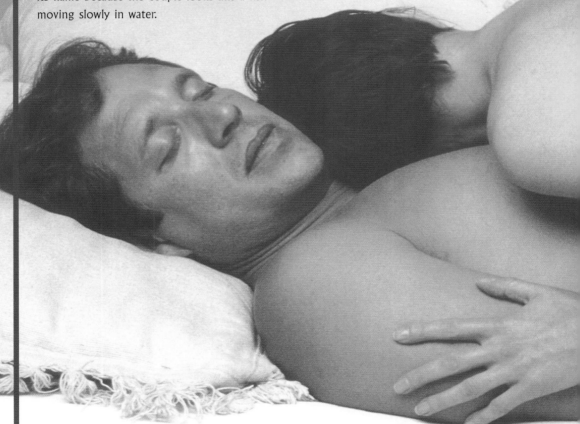

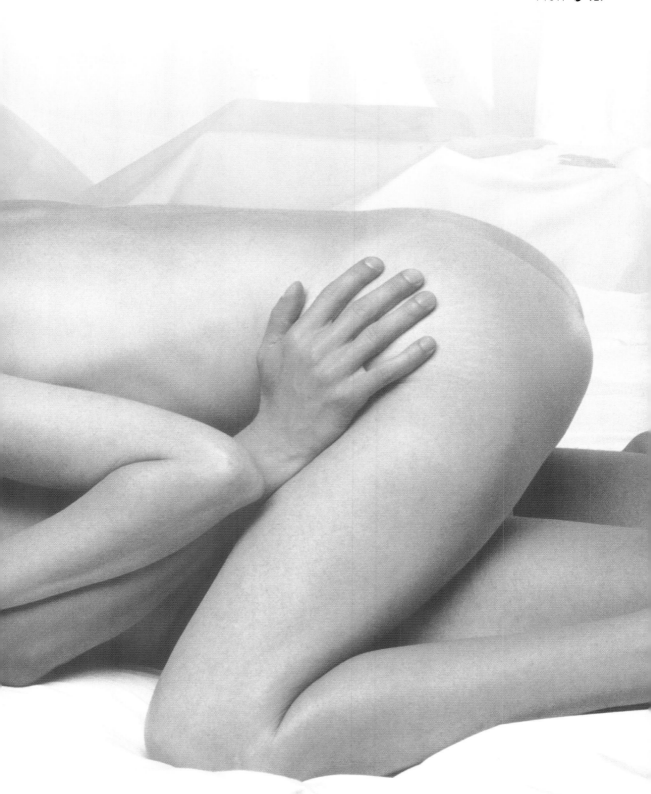

CRANE

HOW-TO The man kneels down and opens his legs, and the woman sits on top of him. The two partners cross their necks. During this move, the man will hold onto the woman's hips and help her gyrate, and the woman will hold onto the man's shoulders or back to further help herself move. The thrusts should begin slowly and shallowly. The thrusts can increase in speed and depth as the woman's vagina grows moister.

ABOUT THE POSITION The Crane enables a woman to move on different angles to direct the penis to different points inside her. According to Lady Xuan, the greater number of points touched, the more health-promoting the lovemaking.

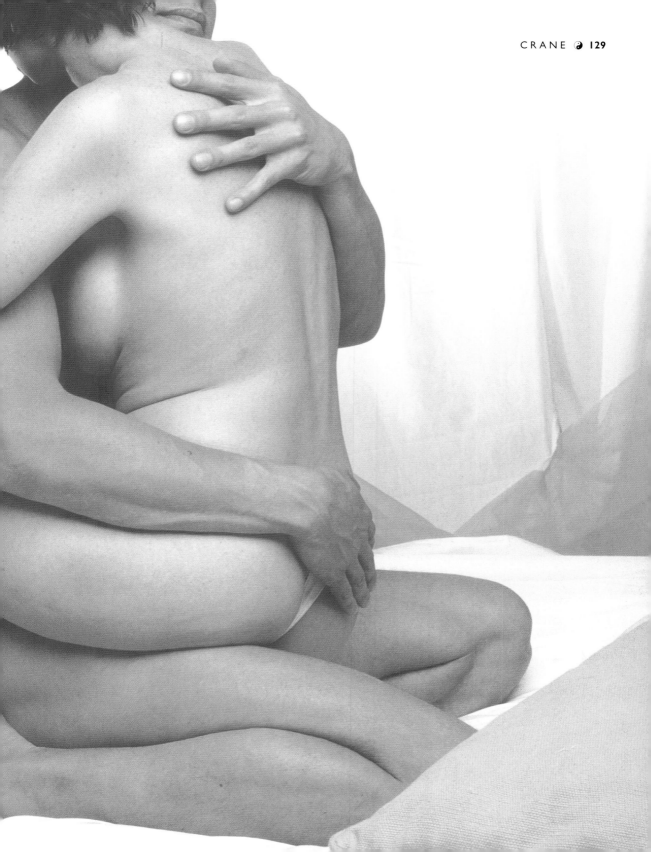

HEALING
BY THE
LOVER —
THE
WOMAN'S
ROLE

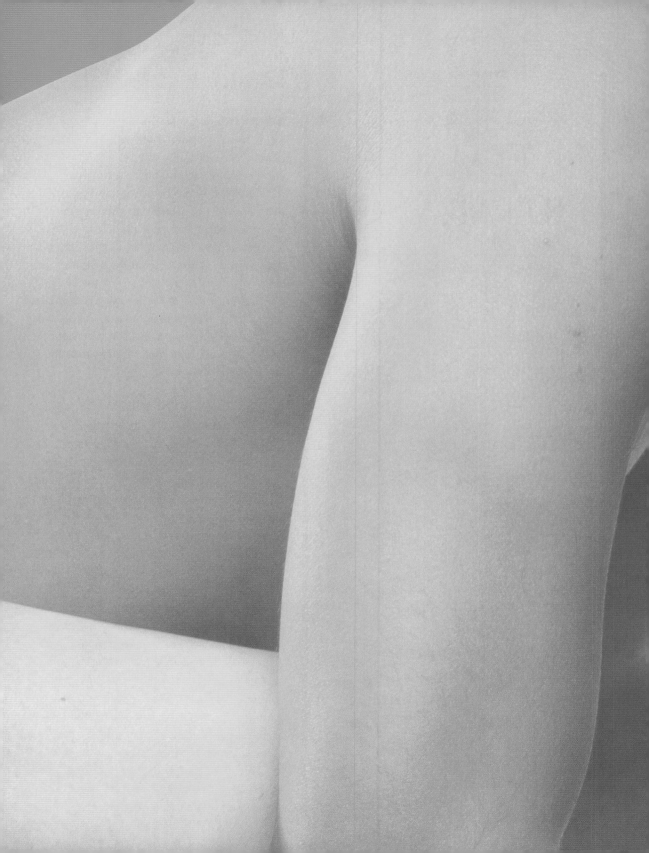

CHAPTER SEVEN

FEMALE PREPARATION

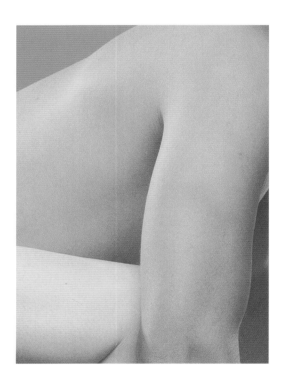

WESTERNERS ARE VERY
COMFORTABLE WITH THE
IDEA OF EXERCISING THEIR BODIES
AND MINDS. BUT MANY ARE NOT
FAMILIAR WITH THE CONCEPT OF
SEXUAL EXERCISE.

DAILY EXERCISE

WE exercise our bodies with gym workouts, hikes, jogs around the park, in-line skating. We exercise our minds with word games, books, classes, a favorite hobby. But what about sexual exercise? While the concept is unfamiliar in Western society, it is well-known in China—and with good reason. When a woman is sexually strong, she is able to control her own orgasms and those of her partner. This in turn leads to more enjoyable lovemaking. Sexual strength is also necessary to perform any of the healing exercises in Chapter 8. The following daily exercises are designed to strengthen the anal, vaginal, and pelvic muscles. You may see subtle results at the end of one week, with maximum results at the end of three months.

GETTING YIN FROM YANG

Five thousand years ago lived Xi Wang Mu, the mythical Queen of the Western Kingdom of the Taoists. Known historically as the Western Kingdom Queen, it is said that she appeared younger every single time she had sex while her partner usually looked exhausted. In fact, when the Western Kingdom Queen was 50 years old, she looked 20. Her secret? She knew how to get yin from yang.

Getting yin from yang fell out of favor during the female-repressive Qin dynasty (221 to 207 B.C.). However, the technique is often discussed in sexual manuals written before this period. This ancient practice allows women to retain their own sexual energy while also gaining healing energy from their partner. At the heart of the technique is orgasm control for both partners. Taoists believe that when a woman climaxes at the same time as her partner, her uterus is able to pull the chi up into her body. Once in the body, the chi moves up the spine to the woman's brain, where it works its regenerative powers. (After receiving a partner's energy, some women notice that their body feels lighter and stronger, and things around them appear brighter.) Getting yin from yang isn't difficult, although it does require that a woman maintain full control of her body, her genitals, her breath, and her partner's responses. To achieve this control, daily sexual exercise is essential.

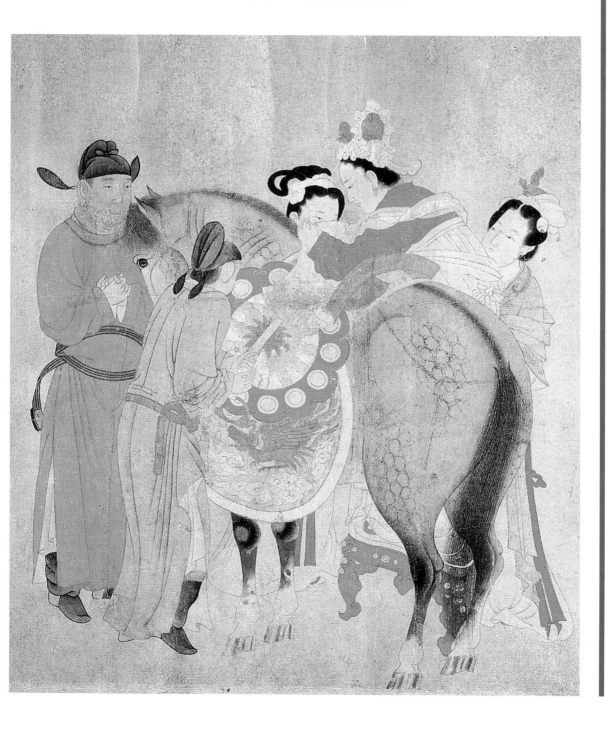

FIRST LEVEL EXERCISES

F IRST level sexual exercises are standing exercises, designed to be done in the following numerical sequence.

Rotating the hips should be done slowly and carefully.

Avoid locking the knees.

LI-STYLE EXERCISES

EXERCISE 1
Stand with legs one foot apart. Simultaneously contract the vaginal and sphincter muscles. Hold for five seconds and release. Perform ten times.

EXERCISE 2
Stand with legs one foot apart. Contract the abdominal, hip, gluteus, and quadriceps muscles. While these muscles are contracted, move hips clockwise. Relax muscles. Perform ten times. Repeat Exercise 1, but perform five times.

EXERCISE 3
Stand with legs one foot apart. Contract the abdominal, hip, gluteus, and quadriceps muscles. While these muscles are contracted, move hips counter-clockwise. Relax muscles. Perform ten times. Repeat Exercise 1, but perform five times.

SECOND LEVEL EXERCISES

TANG-STYLE EXERCISES

EXERCISE 1
Lay face-up on a bed or the floor with knees bent and feet spread one foot apart. Using the thighs, the hamstrings, and the gluteus muscles, slowly lift the hips from the bed. The arms should be lying comfortably at your sides. Continue lifting until the hips cannot go any further. Hold for five seconds. Slowly return to original position. Perform 20 to 50 times, depending on your fitness level.

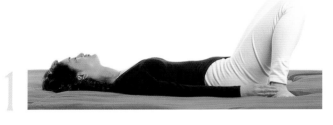

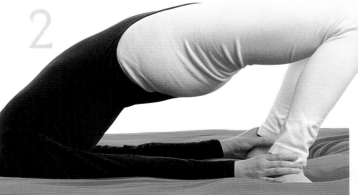

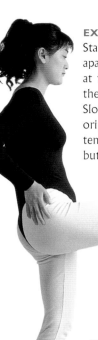

EXERCISE 4

Stand with legs one foot apart. Bend the right leg at the knee and slowly lift the knee toward the chest. Slowly lower the leg to its original position. Perform ten times. Repeat Exercise 1, but perform five times.

EXERCISE 6

Stand with legs one foot apart. Bend the left leg at the hip and slowly lift it sideways until a 90-degree angle is created. Slowly lower the leg to its original position. Perform ten times. Repeat Exercise 1, but perform five times.

If you can not lift your let to a 90-degree angle, just do your best.

EXERCISE 5

Stand with legs one foot apart. Bend the left leg at the knee and slowly lift the knee toward the chest. Slowly lower the leg to its original position. Perform ten times. Repeat Exercise 1, but perform five times.

EXERCISE 7

Stand with legs one foot apart. Bend the right leg at the hip and slowly lift it sideways until a 90-degree angle is created. Slowly lower the leg to its original position. Perform ten times. Repeat Exercise 1, but perform five times.

EXERCISE 2

Lay face-up on a bed or the floor with knees bent and feet spread one foot apart. From the waist, slowly raise the knees toward the chest. The arms should be lying comfortably at your sides. Continue lifting until the knees cannot go any further. Hold for five seconds. Slowly return to original position. Perform 20 to 50 times, depending on your fitness level.

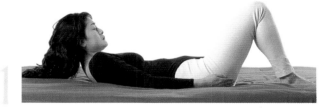

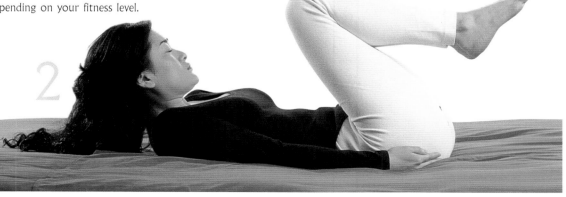

EXERCISE 3

The starting position for this exercise is identical to the ending position of Tang-Style Exercise 3: Legs, hips, lower back, mid-back, and shoulders should all be rolled toward the head, the legs should be draped over the head, and the arms held against the sides of the body. From this position, use the stomach muscles to slowly unfurl the legs until they are almost straight. Hold for five seconds before slowly returning to the starting position. Perform 20 to 50 times, depending on your fitness level.

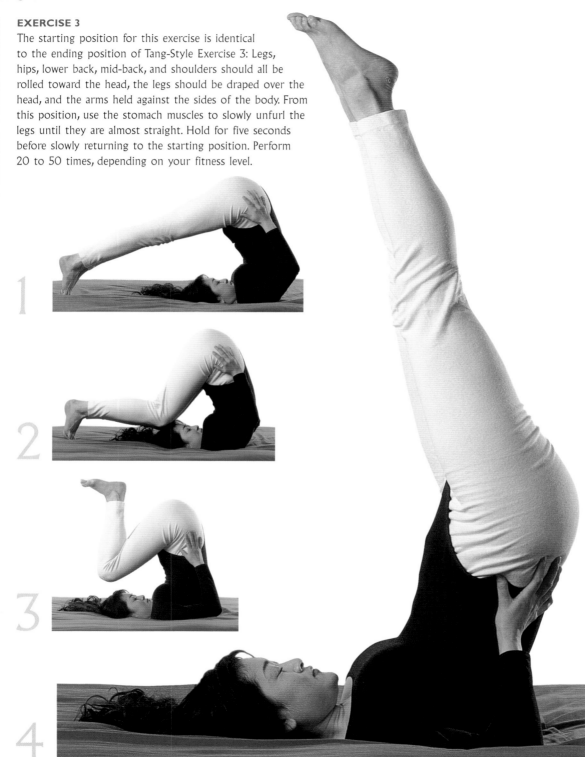

EXERCISE 4

Lay face-up on a bed or the floor with knees bent and feet spread one foot apart. Slowly roll the hips, then lower back, then mid-back, then shoulders, toward the head as if doing a backward somersault. The arms should be held at the sides of the body. Straighten the legs and drape them over the head. Hold for five seconds. Slowly return to original position. Perform 20 to 50 times, depending on your fitness level.

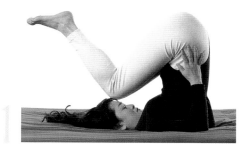

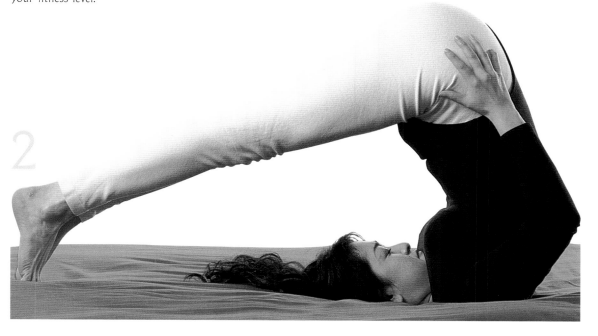

DUN-STYLE EXERCISE

Stand straight with legs one foot apart. Bend arms at the elbows, holding forearms parallel to the floor. Slowly bend at the knees, lowering the body until the hips are level with the knees. Hold for five seconds. If possible, lower the body further until the hips are level with the calves. Slowly return to original position. Perform 20 to 50 times, depending on your fitness level. Note: To help protect the back, be careful to hold the spine straight and use only the thigh, buttock, hip, and abdominal muscles.

JADE BALL EXERCISE

Jade balls are smaller than golf balls and are placed inside the vagina, where they are believed to strengthen the vaginal muscles and increase a woman's sensitivity. Traditionally, a single ball is inserted into the vagina or placed further up in the uterus and left in place for up to an entire day. As a woman gets used to the ball, she may be able to control it, moving it inside her using your vaginal and pelvic muscles. Note: This ancient exercise is not regularly practiced today. A jade ball used currently should have a string attached.

DILDO EXERCISE

To strengthen the entrance of the vagina, many Chinese women use penis-shaped objects called dildos. To use, insert the dildo into the vagina. Leaving the dildo in place, tighten the vaginal muscles around it. Hold for five seconds then loosen the vaginal muscles. Perform 50 times daily. In ancient China, dildos were often fashioned from a stiff flour-and-water dough; in fact, Lady Su recommends a dough dildo in her *Book of Lady Su*.

CHAPTER EIGHT

SEVEN DESTROY

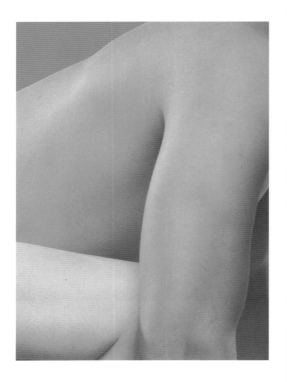

FOR CENTURIES CHINESE TAOISTS
HAVE USED SEX TO HEAL
EVERYTHING FROM MALAISE
TO ABDOMINAL UPSET, FROM
GENERAL FATIGUE TO HEADACHES.

HEALING EXERCISES BY WOMEN

S AY the word 'sex' and chances are either 'fun' or 'fertility' jump to mind. And while recreation and procreation are both terrific reasons for having sex, sex can be used for so much more—more specifically, healing. A woman can help heal a man in just this way with sexual positions called Seven Destroy. Designed specifically for women to heal their partners of various ailments, Seven Destroy exercises are named after the seven types of conditions they are said to destroy.

A note on the following exercises: When using sex as a healing aid, it is suggested that orgasm be withheld. The Chinese believe that female and male ejaculate liquids carry precious health-boosting chi away from the body. A person who is unwell cannot afford to lose any of this vital chi, therefore all exercises should be performed to the point before orgasm, no further. Should you or your partner feel ready to climax, stop the exercise. While orgasm leaches this chi from the body, Taoists believe that the actual sex act increases levels of body chi and helps it to flow more efficiently. Therefore, having sex without orgasm allows you and your partner to build chi without giving any of it away.

SEXUAL CURES

The following exercises describe common male symptoms, then provide a sexual cure that a woman can perform to heal her partner. You will notice that repetition numbers are not given here because every woman is different: The exercises are to be performed until the woman's genitals are well-lubricated. As many times as the exercise must be repeated in order to ensure lubrication is considered one set. Anyone who has ever lifted weights is familiar with the concept: A set consists of one move that is repeated a prescribed number of times. After the set is performed there is a rest period before another set of the same move is performed. The following exercises suggest nine sets spaced over the course of a day. According to ancient prescriptions, these nine sets should be done every day for ten days. Sex several times a day may have been possible for royalty and other elite of ancient China, but it may be impossible for the modern couple with work, family, and personal commitments. Therefore, use the set numbers as a guideline; doing as many sets as you can is better than doing none at all.

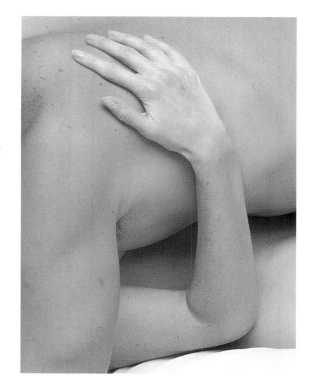

For exercises men can use to heal women, see Eight Benefits, beginning on page 166.

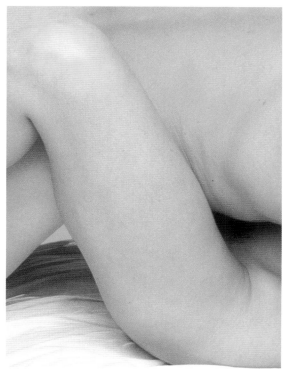

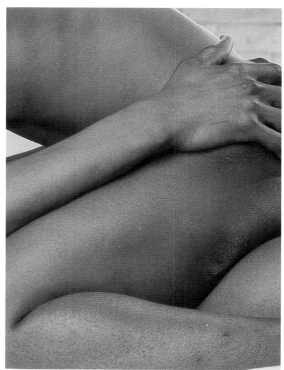

BLOCK THE CHI • JUE CHI 保 留 絕 氣

CONDITION A man with a low libido is a man who consistently does not want to make love. The Chinese believe that this is a sign of low chi, which, with time, can produce profuse sweating and possible heart conditions.

CURE HOW-TO The woman lies on her back with her legs shoulder-width apart. The man kneels below her hips, facing her. The woman then raises her legs and wraps them around her partner's waist and moves her genitals back and forth against her partner's genitals. This should be continued until the woman's genitals are wet. There is penetration.
NOTE: Though he may be tempted to press against his partner or even insert his penis, it is important that the man remain still.

FREQUENCY Traditionally, couples practice Jue Chi nine times a day for ten days.

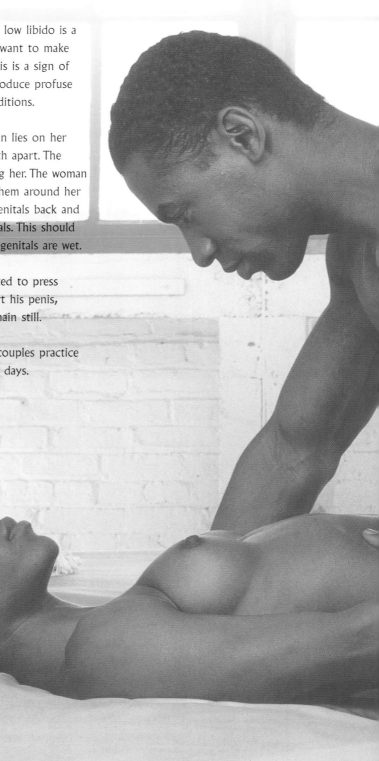

FOCUS BOX

Because of the direct genital contact prescribed by Jue Chi, the position is especially provocative for the man, who is required to do nothing but kneel and watch his partner do the sexual work. This may be difficult at first and the man will be tempted to engage in intercourse. It is a temptation that should be resisted. In order for Jue Chi to work, it is important that the man become sexually excited enough to boost his chi levels, but not so excited that he climaxes and loses the chi that has just been produced.

SPILL THE LIQUID • YI JING 溢 精

CONDITION Sometimes a man's mind wants more orgasms than his body can comfortably produce. When this occurs, the frequent loss of semen drains his chi, resulting in weakness, irritability, and fatigue. Furthermore, lung problems can develop when chi is overdrawn, leaving a man susceptible to coughing, dry mouth, and hot flashes. If a man with this condition drinks alcohol, he may experience painful breathing and he may have trouble standing.

CURE HOW-TO The woman lies on her back with her legs shoulder-width apart. The man kneels below the woman's hips and inserts his penis two inches only, then places his arms on each side of his partner's head. The woman then wraps her legs around the man's waist and swings her hips right and left until her genitals are wet. When this happens, the man should remove his penis.

FREQUENCY Traditionally, couples practice Yi Jing nine times a day for ten days.

FOCUS BOX

Although physically easy, Yi Jing can be an especially challenging position for many couples because the exercise requires a man to insert his penis no more than two inches into his partner's vagina—a feat made more difficult when the woman begins to move back and forth and he is required to hold his penis in place.

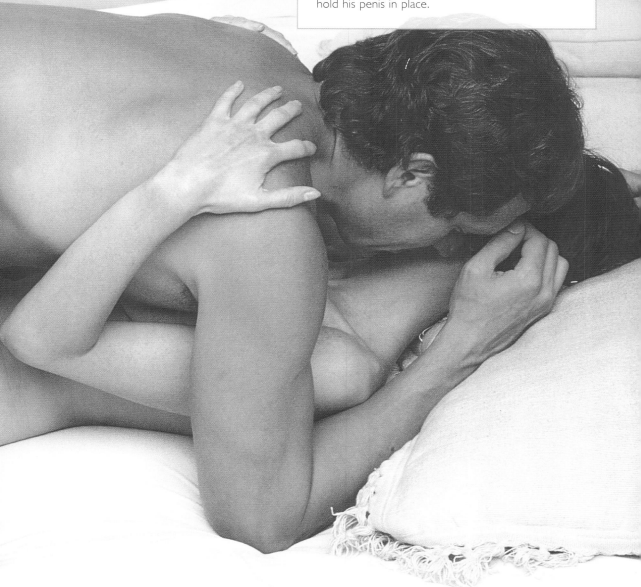

CONDITION If a man frequently has sex after eating, the Chinese believe that he risks harming his spleen. This is because undigested food may cause the stomach to weigh against the spleen. Also, after eating, the body's chi congregates in the stomach to aid digestion, not leaving enough chi to form strong semen.

CURE HOW-TO The woman lies on her back, with her legs shoulder-width apart. Facing her, the man kneels below her hips. She wraps her legs over the man's hips and gently moves her body up and down over the man's genitals and lower abdomen. It is imperative that the man remain completely still while the woman does this. When the woman's genitals become wet she can stop.

FREQUENCY Traditionally, couples practice Duo Mai nine times a day for ten days.

FOCUS BOX

Taoists believe that Duo Mai is a powerful tool to help men who suffer from digestive irregularities. There are other helpful measures men can take to help overcome this type of condition. Chinese tradition maintains that certain foods, such as soybeans and other soy foods, are particularly beneficial to the digestive system, as is a glass of warm water drunk upon waking each morning.

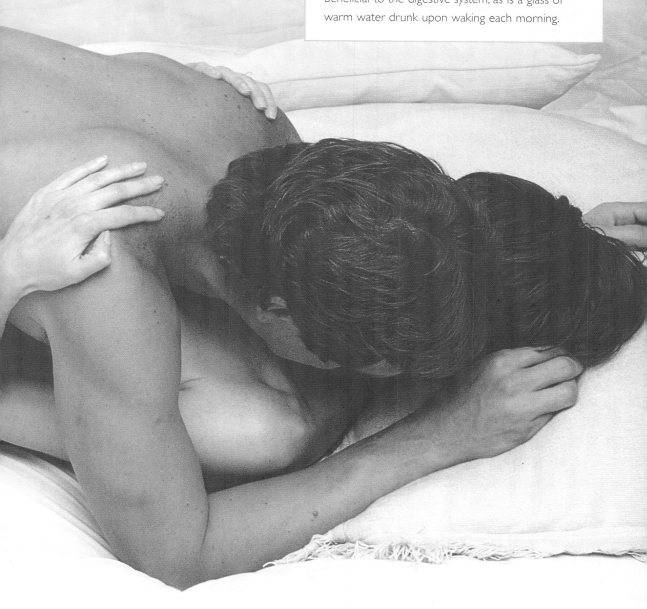

LOSING CONTROL OF CHI • CHI XIE

CONDITION Men who routinely have sex immediately after a sweaty round of exercise or physical labor often develop dry mouth and aches in the lower part of the abdomen. When the body is wet with perspiration, chi travels to the skin to help preserve precious body heat. This leaves the rest of the body with weak chi, which is manifested in abdominal aches and a parched mouth.

CURE HOW-TO The man lies on his back with legs straight and slightly apart. Facing her partner, the woman lowers herself onto the man's hips and straddles them. Her genitals should be directly beneath her partner's testicles. While the man lies still, the woman rotates her hips clockwise, continuing until her genitals are wet.

FREQUENCY Traditionally, couples practice Chi Xie nine times a day for ten days.ten days.

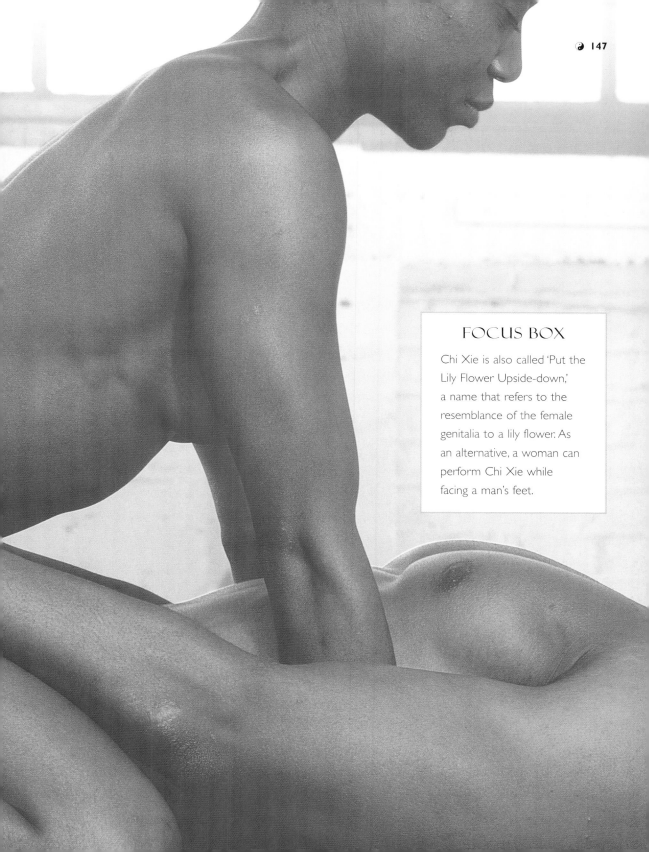

FOCUS BOX

Chi Xie is also called 'Put the
Lily Flower Upside-down,'
a name that refers to the
resemblance of the female
genitalia to a lily flower. As
an alternative, a woman can
perform Chi Xie while
facing a man's feet.

LONG TERM INNER ORGAN DISEASE • JI GUAN 長期內臟病

CONDITION According to Chinese healing beliefs, when a man has sex while afflicted with a condition that affects one of his internal organs, he can suffer from fatigue, general weakness, and even bone aches. A body that is already exhausted from an illness will become even more exhausted with orgasm.

CURE HOW-TO The man lies face-up with his legs slightly apart. The woman faces the man's feet and lowers herself onto his hips. Bending forward at the waist, the woman places her hands on either side of the man's calves to support her weight. The woman gently moves her body up and down over the man's genitals and lower abdomen until her genitals are wet.

FREQUENCY Traditionally, couples practice Ji Guan nine times a day for ten days.

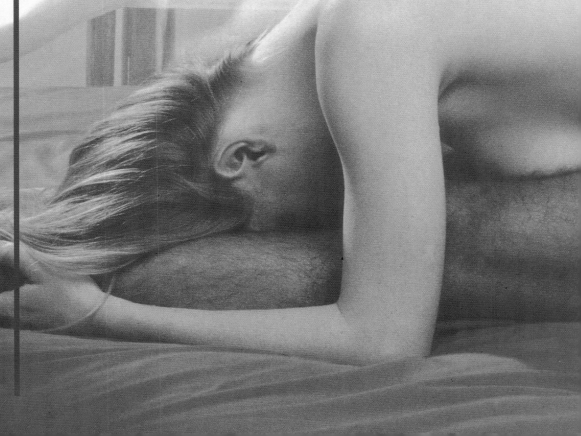

FOCUS BOX

If an ill man does not have a partner, the Ji Guan exercise can be performed alone. To do this, the man should remove his clothing and lie on his back. Holding his penis with his hand, he should gently tighten his grip while inhaling deeply. Upon exhaling, he should loosen his grip. This should be done for ten minutes every day for ten days. Note that this is not masturbation. The hand should not slide up or down the length of the penis, nor should orgasm result.

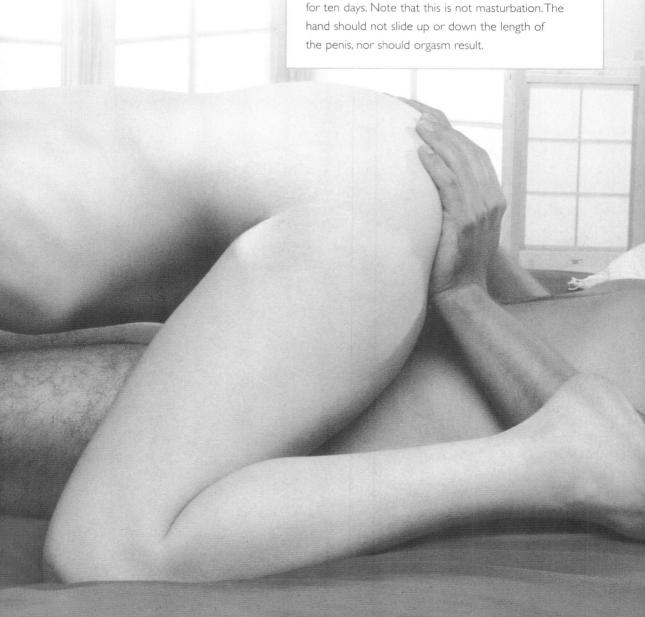

CANNOT COME • BAI BI 百閉

CONDITION When a man has sex or masturbates often, he risks ejaculating too many times. This can greatly diminish the amount of chi in the body, leading to weakness, exhaustion, and even lowered immune system responses, which in turn leaves the body vulnerable to disease.

CURE HOW-TO The man lies face-up with his legs slightly apart. The woman faces the man's feet and lowers herself onto the man's penis. She tightens her vagina's grasp on the penis, and shakes it gently left five times, then right five times, before releasing. There should be no up-and-down motions during this exercise. To shake the penis, a woman can tighten her abdominal and hip muscles, then quickly agitate her hips to the left five times, then to the right five times.

FREQUENCY Traditionally, couples practice Bai Bi nine times a day for ten days.

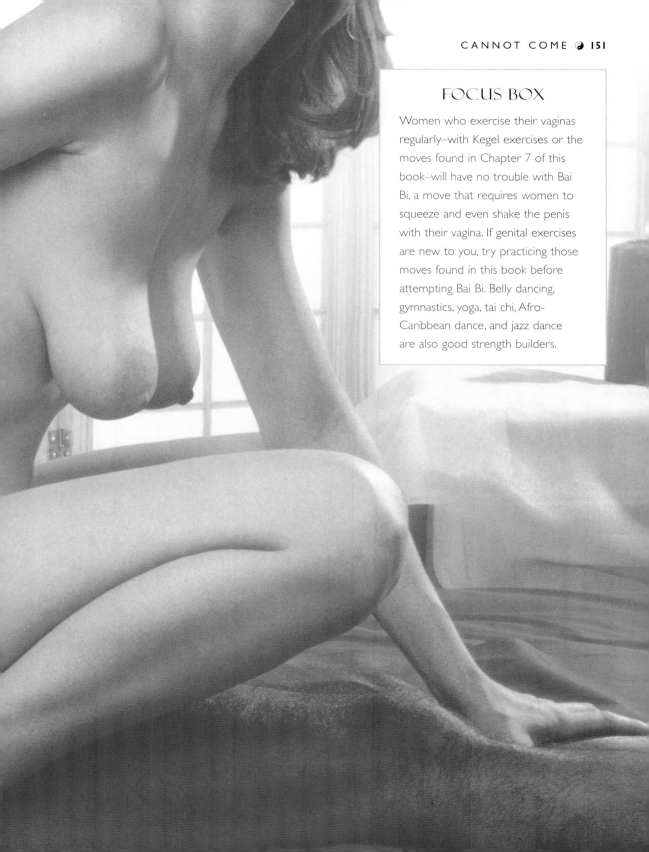

FOCUS BOX

Women who exercise their vaginas regularly—with Kegel exercises or the moves found in Chapter 7 of this book—will have no trouble with Bai Bi, a move that requires women to squeeze and even shake the penis with their vagina. If genital exercises are new to you, try practicing those moves found in this book before attempting Bai Bi. Belly dancing, gymnastics, yoga, tai chi, Afro-Caribbean dance, and jazz dance are also good strength builders.

NOT STOP UNTIL IT IS BLEEDING • XUE JIE 血竭

CONDITION Chinese tradition maintains that having sex when fatigued from intense physical work or exercise can leave the skin shivering, the breath short, the heartbeat weak, the genitals sore, and the groin profusely sweaty. Eventually, the semen may become bloody and a disease of one of the internal organs may develop.

CURE HOW-TO The woman lies on her back with a pillow under her hips and her legs spread shoulder-width apart. The man kneels below his partner's hips and inserts the entire length of his penis. After doing this, the man must hold completely still; he will be tempted to thrust, but must remain stationary. Once the penis is in place, the woman moves her hips left and right. The man should not climax.

FREQUENCY Traditionally, couples practice Xue Jie nine times a day for ten days.

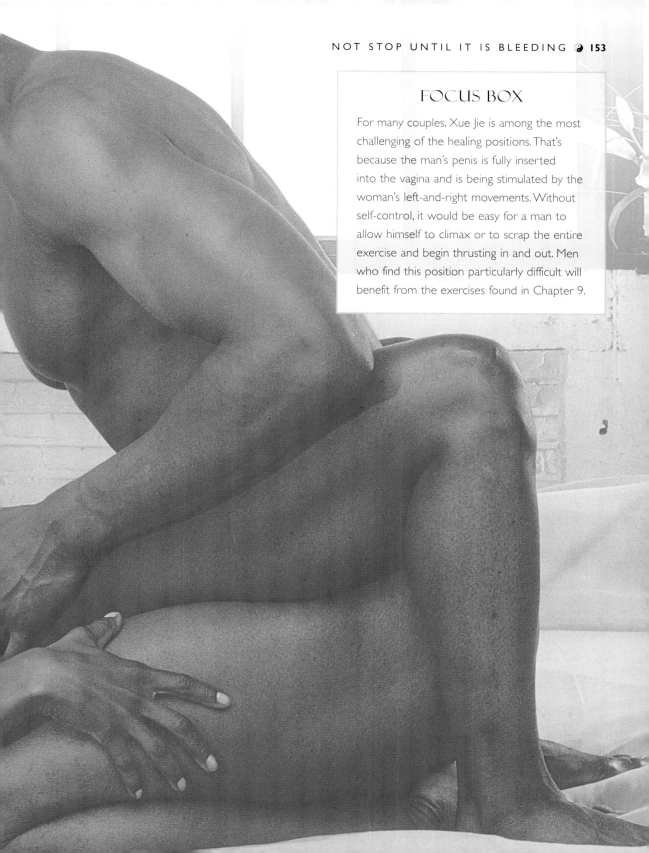

FOCUS BOX

For many couples, Xue Jie is among the most challenging of the healing positions. That's because the man's penis is fully inserted into the vagina and is being stimulated by the woman's left-and-right movements. Without self-control, it would be easy for a man to allow himself to climax or to scrap the entire exercise and begin thrusting in and out. Men who find this position particularly difficult will benefit from the exercises found in Chapter 9.

SEVEN MALE SYMPTOMS TO WATCH FOR

WHEN there is an ailment somewhere in the body, easily visible symptoms occur as indicators of just what, where, and how severe the condition is. When a man develops an inner condition, the woman in his life may be the first one to notice its symptoms:

COLD SWEAT

Also called yin sweat, this indicates a weakness in one or more internal organs. Men with cold sweat are usually healed with rest. If the sweat is particularly profuse, the Chinese advise making an appointment for a general check-up to insure that all organs are functioning properly.

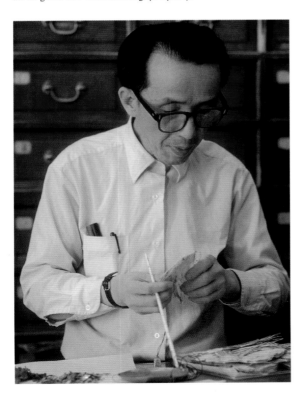

GENERAL WEAKNESS

Also known as yin weakness, this minor condition is usually caused by nothing more than too much physical labor or too little rest. Increased rest is generally all that is required.

THIN, CLEAR SEMEN

In China, doctors commonly examine a man's semen in order to check the prostate's health. Thin, clear semen is seen as a sign of one of many prostate conditions, including prostatitis or prostate cancer.

SCANT SEMEN

When a man releases less than a tablespoon of semen during orgasm, it is a sign that his reproductive organs are being taxed by too-frequent orgasm.

SKIN CONDITION ON OR AROUND THE GENITALS

A rash, pimples, scaly skin, or other skin condition directly on or around the genitals can indicate a yeast or viral infection. Such infections are often symptoms of a sexually transmitted condition and should be examined by a physician.

FREQUENT URINATION

In China, frequent male urination—often accompanied by tenderness, pain, or swelling along the inner legs—is associated with prostatitis. While medication is the common treatment in the West, Chinese doctors use massage to rid the prostate of infection.

IMPOTENCE

In China, impotence is seen as a sign of either a mental condition or a physical illness. If a mild mental condition such as stress is making a man temporarily impotent, his partner can help relax him and help rebuild his energy with one of the Seven Destroy exercises found in Chapter 8. If a more serious mental condition, such as depression, or a physical ailment is the suspected culprit, it is important that a man consult his physician.

PROBLEMATIC SEMEN

THERE may come a time when a man has a health problem that he does not know about. The Chinese believe that a woman can diagnose a man's health condition by noticing the state of his semen. The following signs and symptoms are taken from *The Book of Lady Su.*

SEMEN	POSSIBLE HEALTH CONDITION
Premature in coming	Stress or a nervous system condition
Thin	General weakness or fatigue
Strong smelling	A problem with the tendons
Ejected in a weak stream	A problem with the bones

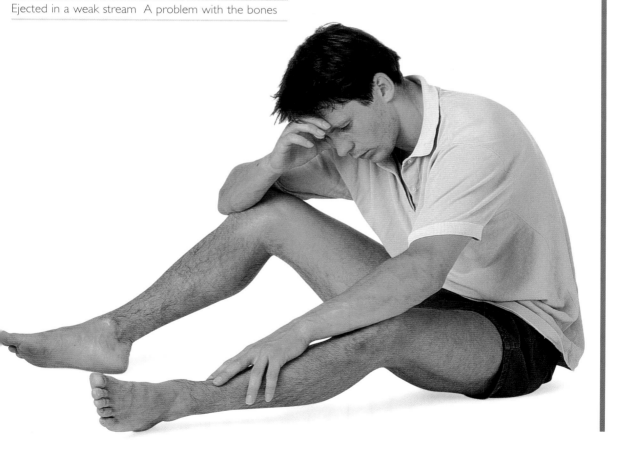

HEALING
BY THE
LOVER –
THE
MAN'S
ROLE

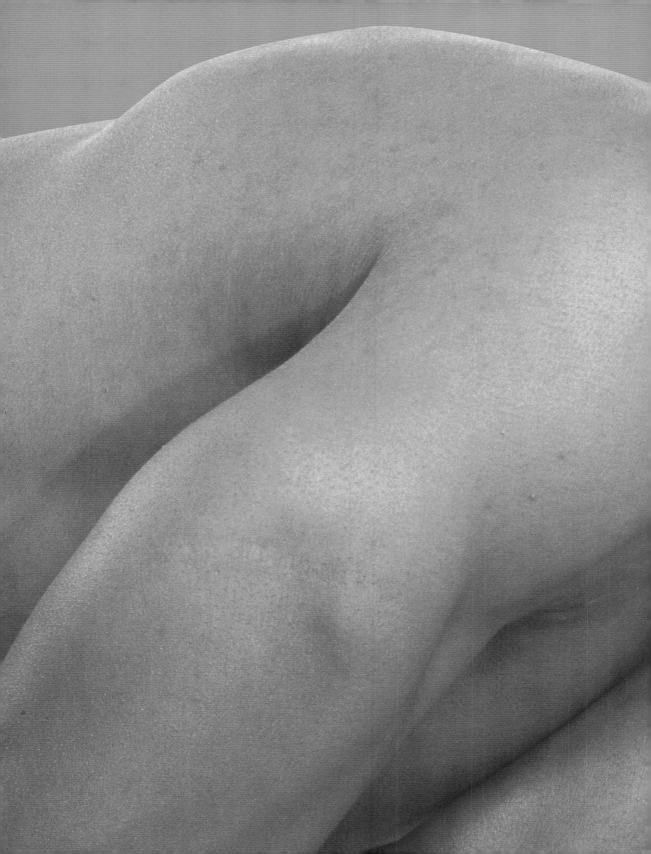

CHAPTER NINE

MALE PREPARATION

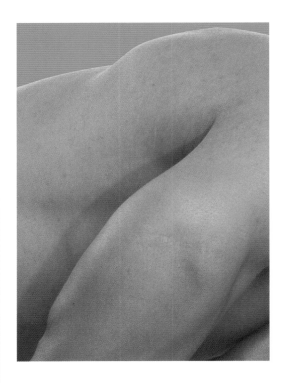

IN CHINA, GOOD SEX DEPENDS
ON A DAILY SET OF MOVEMENTS
THAT HELP MEN DEVELOP SEXUAL
SENSITIVITY AND CONTROL.

EXERCISES FOR MEN

SEX is just like cooking or dancing or singing—a skill that does not require special training. However, like cooking or dancing or singing, sexual technique can be greatly improved with education and practice. It is possible to have sex that is both good—and good for you.

A man who is aware of both his own and his partner's needs and is in control of his sexuality is able to bring pleasure to his partner, sustain an erection, and control his and his partner's orgasms. This in turn leads to more enjoyable and healthful lovemaking. Sexual consciousness and discipline are also necessary for the healing exercises described in Chapter 10.

The following daily exercises are designed to increase a man's sexual intuition as well as strengthen the anal, penile, and pelvic muscles. You may see subtle results at the end of one week, with maximum results at the end of three months.

SEMEN RETENTION–
PRESSURE POINT OF HUI YIN

Hui yin is the acupuncture point midway between the testicles and the anus. This is a popular point for curing prostate problems and helping men to control ejaculation (known in China as 'semen retention'). Semen retention was much practiced by Taoists, who believed that it was a form of energy reabsorption—the withheld semen would draw energy or chi back into the circulatory system and up to the brain, rejuvenating the whole body.

Sun, Si Miao, a doctor and Taoist who lived in A.D. 600, strongly recommended semen retention. He is said to have noted that if a man can manage the energy route in his body, he is able to enjoy sex without ejaculating and also become very youthful.

It is very important to practice this method correctly: It should always be started upon arousal, not when one is about to ejaculate. If practiced too often directly before ejaculation, it is believed that bladder or kidney problems may result, as well as difficulty in ejaculation.

TEN STEPS TO REJUVENATION

The Yellow Emperor tried the semen retention method and reported the following benefits to Lady Su:

After the first time I stopped it,
I gained strength;

After the second time, I felt my eyesight sharpen and my hearing become clearer;

After the third time, I did not feel any sickness;

After the fourth time, I felt my inner organs getting better;

After the fifth time, my blood circulation became smoother;

After the sixth time, my waist grew stronger;

After the seventh time, my hips and my legs got stronger;

After the eighth time, my whole body glowed;

After the ninth time, I felt I could live longer;

And after the tenth time, I feel like I am in heaven.

IRON JADE STALK

In China, a common strengthening exercise involves pushing the erect penis into sand. The exercise is modeled after the Iron Hands, performed by Buddhist Shao Lin monks. The monks flatten their hands, and forcefully push them into the sand, fingertips first. Once the hand is submerged up to the wrist, it is quickly withdrawn, then immediately plunged back into the sand. This is repeated a hundred or more times and is said to strengthen hands so well that they can chop through wood and brick. To try the Iron Jade Stalk, fill a wide bowl with clean sand. Sit the bowl on a table and plunge an erect penis (covered with a condom) into the sand-filled bowl. Start with 20 plunges daily and work up to one hundred.

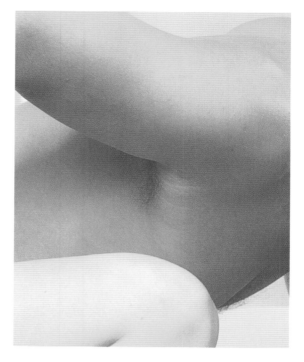

JADE STALK LIFTING

If you have ever done biceps curls, you are familiar with the moves required for Jade Stalk Lifting. Two small objects are tied on each side of a five- to seven-inch piece of rope. These objects can be pieces of fruit, household objects, or actual weights. The rope is then draped over the base of the erect penis. The penis lifts the weights 20 to 50 times daily.
NOTE: One-quarter pound is a good weight to start with. Be careful not to strain or lift too large an amount, the weight can be increased as one's strength grows.

SUN, SI MIAO'S SEMEN RETENTION EXERCISE

Apply pressure to the hui yin point at the beginning of arousal during intercourse. At the same time, close the mouth, keep the eyes open, take a deep breath through the nose and hold it for five to ten seconds, tightening the stomach and buttocks muscles. Exhale slowly through the nose, press the tongue on the roof of the mouth, and tighten the teeth—feel the energy flowing back into the body. This exercise will improve a man's endurance and energy level.
NOTE: A woman can try this exercise to physically and mentally rejuvenate, omitting the first step and following the remaining instructions.

A VARIETY OF THRUSTS

ANCIENT Taoists and Lama Buddhists believed in using a combination of shallow and deep thrusts to create sexual variety, prolong sexual pleasure, and help create health-supportive sex. A shallow thrust involves inserting the penis two inches into the vagina, then pulling it completely out before inserting it again. A deep thrust requires submerging the entire penis into the vagina, then pulling it out completely before re-inserting it. Popular combinations are:

- Eight shallow and five deep
- Five shallow and three deep
- Nine shallow and six deep
- Ten shallow and four deep
- Six shallow and two deep
- Four shallow and one deep
- Ten shallow and seven deep

COMMON SEX-SENSE

Most cultures have sexual rules of conduct that ensure a pleasurable, healthy experience for both sexual partners. In addition to following detailed rules regarding when, where, and how to have sex, the Chinese have strong beliefs about forcing a partner to have sex. In China, verbally or physically coercing a partner who is 'not in the mood' is said to create an erratic flow of chi in the demanding partner's body. On a physical level, a person who does not want sex does not produce the chi needed for healthy sex and instead drains the chi from his or her more amorous partner.

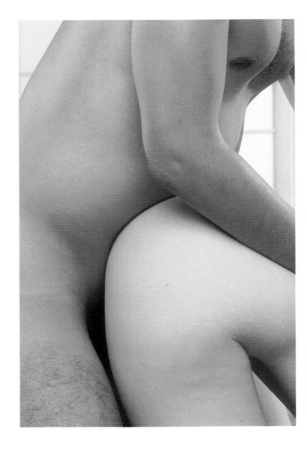

WHY RESIST ORGASM?

For many Westerners, especially men, sex and orgasm are nearly synonymous: What good is the first without the second? The Chinese see things a bit differently: They believe that sex builds chi in the body while orgasm leaches chi. That is not to say that Chinese men never have orgasm; healthy men with healthy partners do enjoy sexual climax. However, there are instances—when practicing the Seven Destroy or Eight Benefits, or when feeling unwell—where Chinese men practice orgasm-free sex as a way to build their and their partner's energy levels.

HOW OFTEN A MAN SHOULD HAVE AN ORGASM

How often you reach orgasm is a matter of personal preference, but having some guidelines may help. According to Chinese thought, a person's age and overall health are important factors in determining the ideal frequency of intercourse. For instance, a young or healthy man can withstand the rigors of frequent orgasm, while an elderly man or someone who is unwell can be weakened by too-frequent orgasm.

Notice that the following charts refer to orgasm only. According to Taoist healers, a man need not forgo sex, but simply limit the amount of chi-disrupting orgasm he experiences. As long as a man doesn't climax, frequent sex is fine. These charts were devised by various Chinese sex experts and may differ in advice. Use them as general guidelines.

LADY SU'S ORGASM FREQUENCY GUIDELINES

Age	Frequency
20	twice a day if healthy, once a day if unwell
30	once a day if healthy, once every 2 days if unwell
40	once every 3 days if healthy, once every 4 days if unwell
50	once every 5 days if healthy, once every 10 days if unwell
60	once every 10 days if healthy, once every 20 days if unwell

PENG ZU'S ORGASM FREQEUNCY GUIDELINES

Age	Frequency
20	once every 2 days
30	once every 3 days
40	once every 10 days
50	once every 15 days
60	once every 30 days

TRADITIONAL SEASONAL ORGASM GUIDELINES

The Chinese believe that the body is strongest in the spring, weakest in the winter. The following numbers are ancient suggestions that apply to healthy middle-aged men.

Season	Frequency
Spring	once every 3 days
Summer	once every 15 days
Fall	once every 15 days
Winter	once every 30 days

FIVE SOUNDS OF A WOMAN

SEX that is both pleasurable and health-supportive requires sensitivity to a partner's needs and readiness. Because a woman's arousal isn't as obvious as a man's, many men have trouble gauging their partner's excitement. To determine their partner's readiness, Chinese men listen for the Five Sounds of a Woman.

SIGH

When a woman first begins to grow aroused, the Chinese say the chi on her skin makes her sigh. At this stage, a man should concentrate on foreplay.

HARD BREATHING

When the chi reaches the inner organs, a woman's arousal increases and her breathing becomes harder. This is when a man can begin intercourse.

SLOW, TIRED, SAD SOUND

As intercourse continues, a woman may look and sound tired but her senses are extremely sharp. According to the Chinese, this is because chi has infused her nervous system.

BEGGING SOUND

As the woman nears orgasm, she may be physically exhausted and may make a series of short, breathy noises. Though she is unable to move her body, her senses have become even sharper. At this stage, the Chinese say the woman's chi is flowing between the mind of pleasure and the mind of suffering, a point near ecstasy.

SCREAMING SOUND

In the West, screaming is associated with orgasm. It is no different in China, where a woman who is climaxing may make a series of loud, sharp cries.

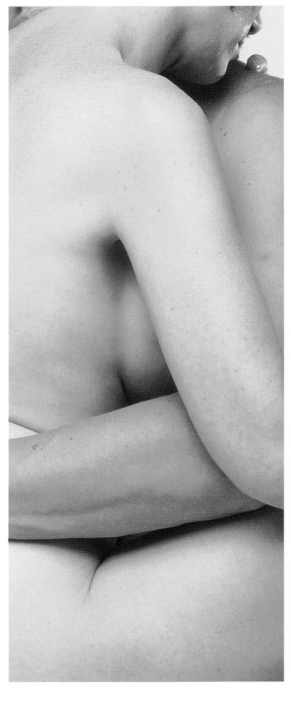

During climax a woman's chi is extremely strong and is flowing out of the vagina, where it enters her partner or leaves her body.

FIVE DESIRES OF A WOMAN

IN addition to The Five Sounds of a Woman, men who are trying to gauge their partner's arousal can also study The Five Desires of a Woman. These are physical signs that the Taoists believed to be indications of how excited a woman's body is during intercourse.

YI (MIND DESIRE)

Breathing gets more rapid. The Chinese believe that this stage is ruled by the mind, which desires sexual contact.

YIN (YIN DESIRE)

The mouth and nostrils open wide. This stage represents an accumulation of yin energy in a woman's body. Note that in Chinese, 'yin' can mean the woman's body itself or the yin energy of both partners.

JING (SPIRIT DESIRE)

Passion drives a woman to press her body against her partner's; she may even hold the man tightly between her legs. At this point, a woman's sexual energy has entered—and controls—her spirit.

XIN (HEART DESIRE)

A woman begins to perspire heavily. Some women may soak the sheets under them or their clothing. When a woman reaches heart desire, the Chinese believe she is physically ready for climax.

KUAI (FAST DESIRE)

The body is rigid; eyes are closed. Fast desire is the state a woman enters as she climaxes. It is during fast desire that a woman releases chi into her vagina, where it can be taken up by her partner or emptied from the body. The name comes from the quick movements the man must make.

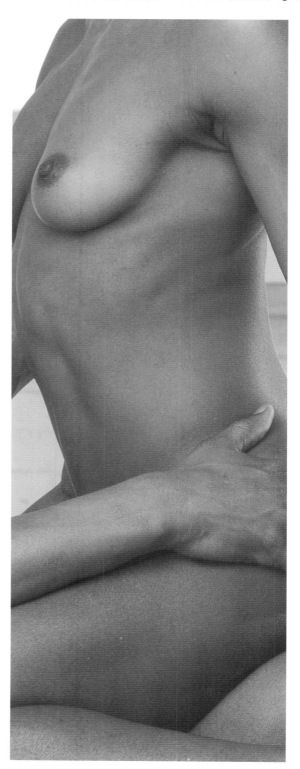

TEN MOVES FROM A WOMAN

I N *The Book of Lady Su*, The Yellow Emperor asks, 'How can I tell if my partner is enjoying herself?'

Lady Su tells him to watch for the Ten Moves from a Woman. These movements show a woman's progression through desire, arousal, and orgasm. It should be noted that every woman displays slightly different signs of excitement; therefore, the Ten Moves from a Woman are designed as a general guide to help men.

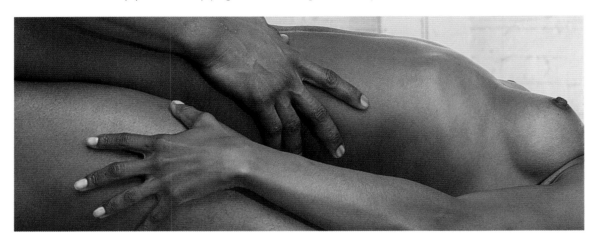

1 The woman holds herself against the man, touching her genitals to his.

2 She stretches her legs and hips to rub against the man with the upper part of her genitals.

3 She opens her legs to welcome the man.

4 The woman's shoulders move, which indicates that the chi is flowing freely through her body, encouraging it to move.

5 She bends her legs and digs the heels of her feet into the bed, raising her waist to ease the man's penis deeper inside her. Or she wraps her legs around her partner's waist to help the man penetrate her more deeply.

6 She holds her legs tight. Her genitals produce liquid.

7 She shifts her hips to get the penis even deeper inside her.

8 She bends her body and pulls the man closer, indicating that she is close to orgasm.

9 She stretches her limbs their full length and holds them stiff during orgasm, then relaxes them as she nears the end of her climax.

10 In some women, liquid emerges from the vagina after orgasm.

GETTING YANG FROM YIN

IN the simplest terms, yin represents female and yang represents male. Yet humans—regardless of their gender—are made up of both yin energy and yang energy. Therefore, a man who is short on yang energy can get some from his partner through intercourse. This ancient practice—called getting yang from yin—allows men to retain their own sexual energy while also gaining healing energy from their partner. At the heart of the technique is orgasm control for both partners. Taoists believe that when a man climaxes at the same time as his partner, his penis can pull the chi in the woman's vaginal secretions up into his own body. Once in the body, the chi moves up the spine to the man's brain, where it works its regenerative powers. (After receiving a partner's energy, some men notice their body feels lighter and stronger and things around them appear brighter.) Getting yang from yin isn't difficult, although it does require that a man be fully aware of his partner's sexual state and in full control of his own body. To achieve this control, daily sexual exercise is essential.

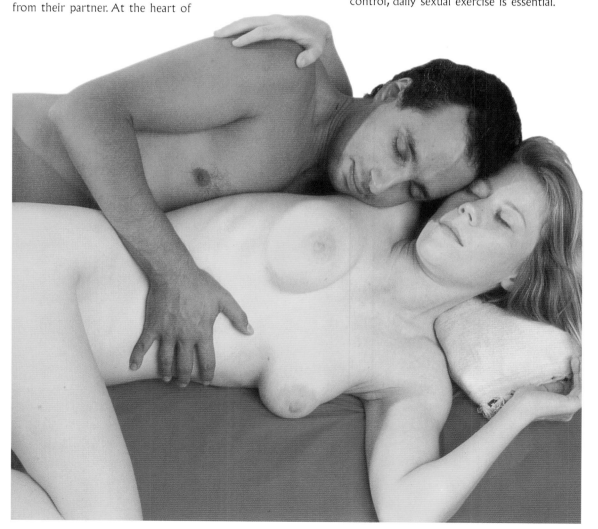

☯

EIGHT
BENEFITS

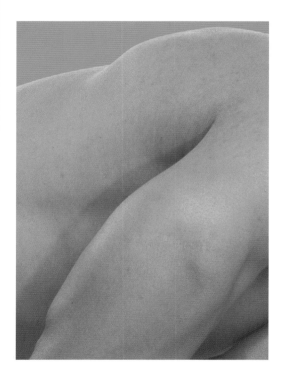

DESIGNED SPECIFICALLY FOR MEN
TO HEAL THEIR PARTNERS
OF VARIOUS AILMENTS,
EIGHT BENEFITS ARE NAMED AFTER
THE EIGHT TYPES OF CONDITIONS
HELPED BY THE EXERCISES.

HEALING EXERCISES BY MEN

SEX. In Western societies the word most often refers to pleasure or procreation. While Chinese Taoists also use intercourse for fun and fertility, they don't stop there. For them, sex is considered a powerful form of healing. For centuries they have used sex to heal everything from malaise to menstrual pain, from general fatigue to headaches.

A man can help heal a woman in just this way with sexual positions called Eight Benefits. These entries describe common female symptoms then provide a sexual exercise that a man can perform to heal his partner. Because the Chinese believe in vaginal reflexology, which means that different areas of the vagina are associated with specific corresponding organs, each position is designed to heal a particular problem by stimulating the corresponding part of the vagina. Fingers and dildos are not recommended. A finger is not usually long enough to reach a certain spot and a dildo can be too hard or cold for the healing process.

Though the Eight Benefits requires the man to play the more active role, the woman must be a cooperative partner. Many of the positions require the woman's legs to be bent, opened, or crossed while her waist moves from left to right. The Chinese believe that this combination of leg positions and waist movements improves blood circulation to a woman's organs, improves her muscle strength, and enhances vaginal functioning.

WITHHOLDING ORGASM
When using sex as a healing aid, orgasm should be withheld. The Chinese believe that female and male ejaculate liquids carry precious health-boosting chi away from the body. A person who is unwell cannot afford to lose any of this vital chi, therefore all exercises must be performed to the point just

before orgasm, no further. Should you or your partner feel on the verge of climax, stop the exercise. While orgasm leaches this chi from the body, Taoists believe that the actual sex act increases levels of chi in the body and helps this chi to flow more efficiently. Therefore, having sex without orgasm allows you and your partner to build chi without giving any of it away.

The Eight Benefits are identical to the Seven Destroy in that they are performed in sets. As previously mentioned, a set consists of one move that is repeated a prescribed number of times. After the set is performed there is a rest period before another set of the same move is performed. The following exercises suggest nine sets spaced over the course of a day. This may be impractical due to modern time constraints; therefore, use the set numbers as a guideline—doing as many sets as you can is better than doing none at all.

For exercises women can use to heal men, see Seven Destroy, beginning on page 138.

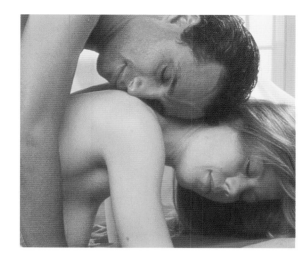

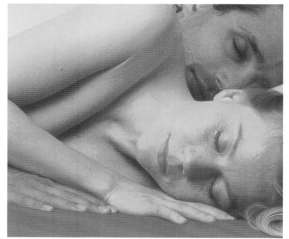

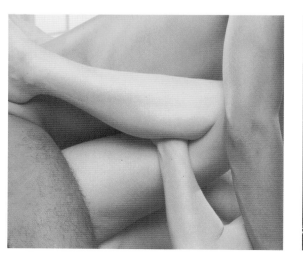

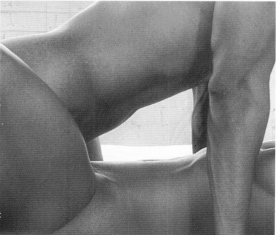

HOLD THE LIQUID · GU JING

CONDITION A woman who suffers from heavy periods may have either too much yin or too much yang in her body; according to Chinese thought both conditions contribute to menstrual irregularities. Chinese usually define food and environment in terms of cold (yin) and hot (yang). A woman who spends too much time in cold temperatures and/or consumes a large quantity of icy foods and beverages (melon, ice cream, soda, iced tea) may develop too much yin and become sluggish and cold. A woman who spends a great deal of time in hot and dry environments and/or eats an overabundance of yang foods and beverages (spicy dishes, chocolate, nuts, and coffee) may develop too much yang and become fidgety and warm. Gu Jing can help either condition by balancing the body's yin and yang.

CURE HOW-TO The couple lies side by side, facing each other. The woman wraps one leg around the man's thigh. He inserts his penis then fully withdraws it, performing this movement a total of 18 times.

FREQUENCY Twice a day for 15 days.

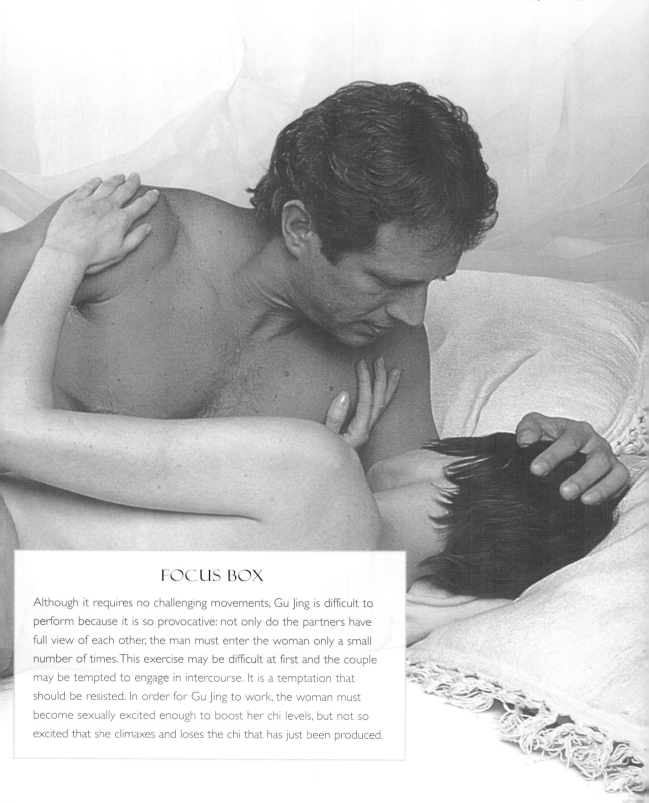

FOCUS BOX

Although it requires no challenging movements, Gu Jing is difficult to perform because it is so provocative: not only do the partners have full view of each other, the man must enter the woman only a small number of times. This exercise may be difficult at first and the couple may be tempted to engage in intercourse. It is a temptation that should be resisted. In order for Gu Jing to work, the woman must become sexually excited enough to boost her chi levels, but not so excited that she climaxes and loses the chi that has just been produced.

CALM THE CHI • AN CHI

好
津

CONDITION When a woman feels nervous, the Chinese say that her chi is jumpy. In other words, her chi is racing erratically through her body. The chi may even travel at different frequencies through different body parts. Stimulating the part of her vagina that corresponds with the nervous system will help soothe her and return her chi to an orderly flow.

CURE HOW-TO Propping a thick pillow under her head, a woman lies on her back with legs bent and spread shoulder-width apart. Facing her, the man lowers himself, placing his arms outside of his partner's arms and holding his weight with both his hands and legs. He inserts his penis then fully withdraws it, performing this movement a total of 27 times.

FREQUENCY Three times a day for 20 days.

FOCUS BOX

An Chi is a good antidote for everyday stress and nervous tension. Other chi-balancing options include full body massage. Like all the positions in this chapter, it is important for a woman to relax and allow herself to receive the benefits of the exercise. For a change, the woman can lie on one of her sides with her partner behind her.

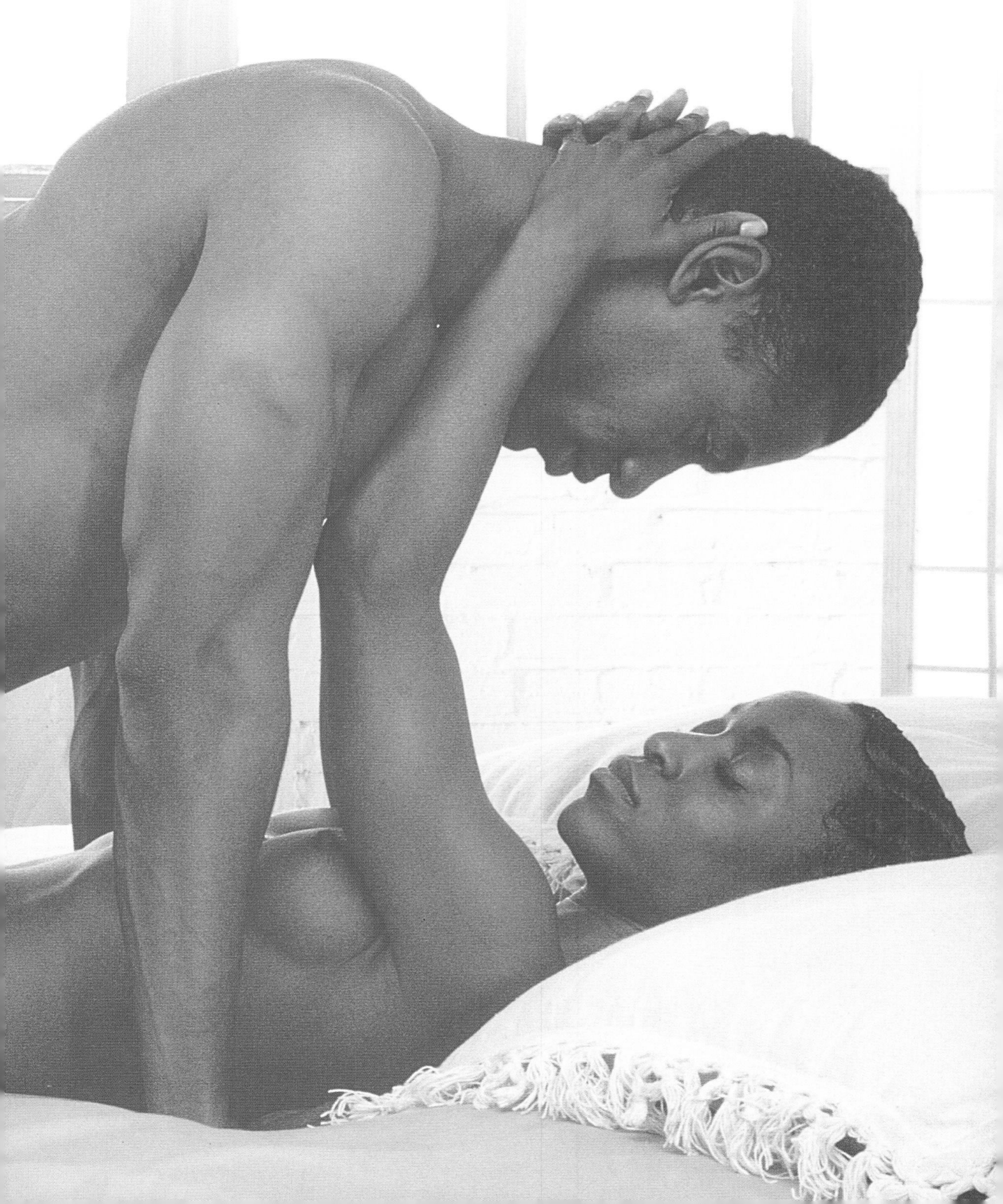

割 臟

BENEFIT THE INNER ORGAN • LI ZANG

CONDITION In China it is believed that when one of the inner organs is not receiving enough chi, it becomes weak. When this happens, a person can feel tired or sluggish, and may become more susceptible to infectious illnesses. Li Zang is not a curative position but a preventative one. It can be used at any time to ensure overall well-being by promoting a smooth flow of chi to all organs.

CURE HOW-TO The woman lies on her right side, facing the outer edge of the bed. She bends her left leg at the knee and raises it until the knee is at hip level. The man lies on his right side directly behind the woman. She reaches her arms behind her and grasps her partnerís hips. Depending on what is most comfortable, the man can reach his arms above his head and hold onto the head of the bed, or he can grasp his partnerís shoulders or hips. He inserts his penis, then withdraws it fully, performing this movement a total of 36 times.

FREQUENCY Four times a day for 20 days.

FOCUS BOX

Li Zang requires a man to perform 36 thrusts, making it difficult for men who suffer from premature ejaculation. Performing the daily penile exercises found in Chapter 9 (page 158) may help a man have more control over his sexuality. In the meantime, any man who feels he is going to climax before finishing the exercise should stop before completing the recommended number of insertions.

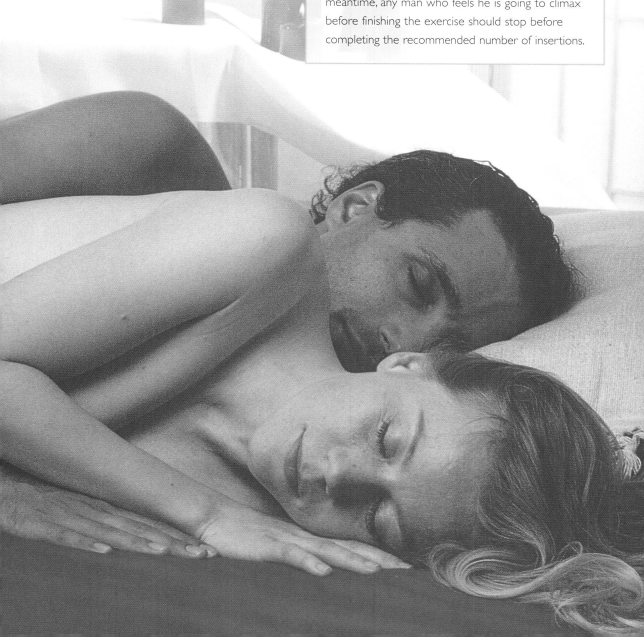

STRENGHTEN THE BONE • QIANG GU

強 骨

CONDITION A woman whose body is stiff and inflexible may suffer from weak, brittle bones. This can be caused when nourishing chi does not adequately reach the bones and joints. Qiang Gu can encourage the flow of chi to the skeletal system and joints.

CURE HOW-TO The woman lies on her left side, the right leg bent, the left leg straight. Facing the bed, the man lowers himself over his partner's right leg and inserts his penis, then withdraws it fully. He performs this movement a total of 45 times. If needed, he can steady himself by clasping the upper edge of the bed.

FREQUENCY Five times a day for 10 days.

FOCUS BOX

Qiang Gu is an awkward position, making it appear more difficult than it is. The key to performing Qiang Gu is for the man to keep his body as straight as possible. Any man who has difficulty thrusting 45 times without climaxing will find that performing the daily penile exercises found in Chapter 9 (page 158) may help him control his sexuality. In the meantime, any man who feels he is going to climax before finishing the exercise should stop before completing the recommended number of insertions.

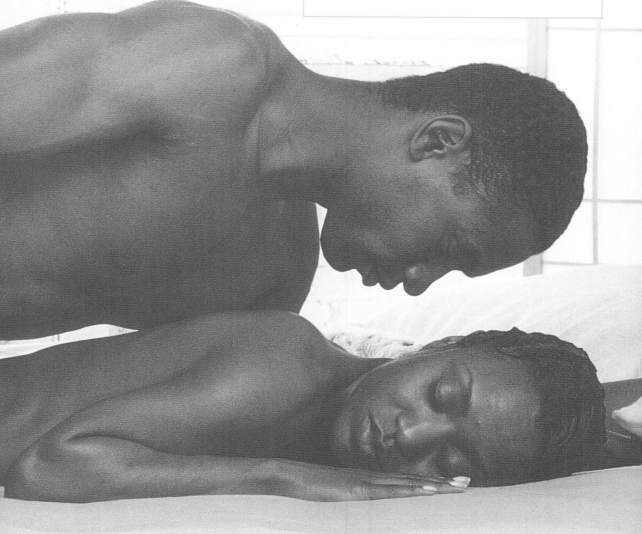

ADJUST THE MERIDIAN & NERVE SYSTEMS • TIAO MAI 調脈

CONDITION According to the Chinese, when a woman encounters stress her chi moves more rapidly through her body's nerve system and along her meridians. The result is a group of symptoms commonly recognized in the West as signs of stress, including irritability, rapid heartbeat, dry mouth, and sweaty palms. Unfortunately, it is difficult to go through a day without encountering at least one or two stressful situations. Fortunately, Tiao Mai can help calm a woman's nerves by slowing the flow of chi to a more normal speed.

CURE HOW-TO The woman lies on her right side with her left leg bent and her right leg straight. Facing the bed, the man lowers himself over his partner's right leg and inserts his penis, then withdraws it fully, performing this movement a total of 54 times. If needed, he can steady himself by clasping the upper edge of the bed.

FREQUENCY Six times a day for 20 days

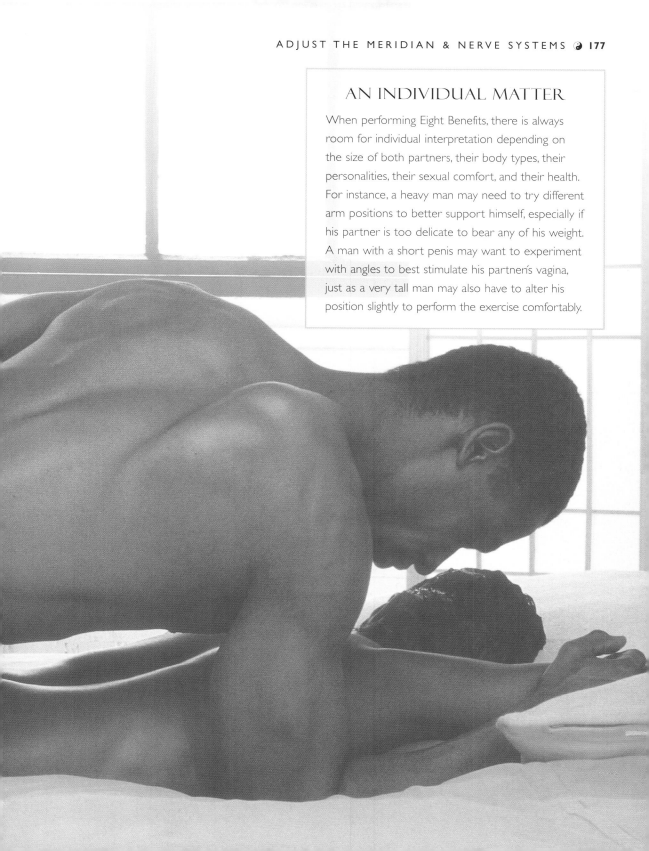

AN INDIVIDUAL MATTER

When performing Eight Benefits, there is always room for individual interpretation depending on the size of both partners, their body types, their personalities, their sexual comfort, and their health. For instance, a heavy man may need to try different arm positions to better support himself, especially if his partner is too delicate to bear any of his weight. A man with a short penis may want to experiment with angles to best stimulate his partner's vagina, just as a very tall man may also have to alter his position slightly to perform the exercise comfortably.

BLOOD STORAGE • XU XUE 蓄血

CONDITION By this point in the book, you are probably aware that balance is the Chinese answer to good health. It is believed that women who enjoy balanced chi are less likely to suffer from irregular menstrual cycles, painful periods, or heavy bleeding. A man can help his partner maintain a balance of chi by performing Xu Xue, which is also said to strengthen the uterine and vaginal muscles.

CURE HOW-TO The man lies on his back. Facing her partner, the woman positions herself over her partner's hips and lowers herself onto his penis. The man grasps her hips and lifts her up three or four inches, then down, performing this movement a total of 63 times. To make this easier for her partner, a woman should relax totally and allow herself to be moved up and down.

FREQUENCY Seven times a day for 10 days

FOCUS BOX

Because it requires that a man move his partner up and down 63 times, Xu Xue is an exercise that requires upper body strength. Any man who doubts his ability to perform Xu Xue may want to perform daily strengthening exercises such as push-ups, pull-ups, and lifting weights.

BENEFIT THE LIQUID · YI YIE 益液

CONDITION In Chinese medicine, the term 'body liquids' refers to any liquid produced by the body, including blood, bile, bone marrow (the Chinese consider marrow a liquid), semen, vaginal fluid, and saliva. When these liquids are manufactured in adequate amounts, the body functions efficiently. If one or more of these liquids is inadequately produced, the Chinese believe that the bodyís immune system can become damaged, leaving a person vulnerable to infectious illnesses. To help his partner maintain good health, a man can perform Yi Yie, an exercise that was designed to help the body generate the necessary body liquids.

CURE HOW-TO The woman lies face down with a pillow under her hips and her legs tightly together. The man kneels behind the woman and places his legs outside his partnerís legs. He inserts his penis, then withdraws it fully, performing this movement a total of 72 times.

FREQUENCY Eight times a day for 10 days.

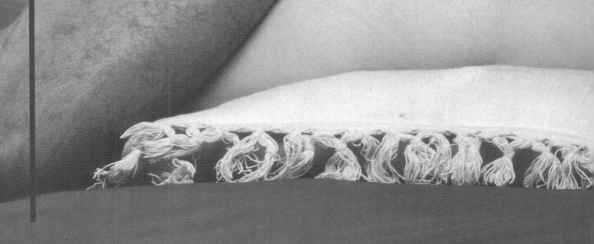

FOCUS BOX

Do you want to help your partner maintain her overall health? Yi Yie is only one of numerous measures you and your partner can take. According to Chinese thought, the best way to create a strong immune system is with daily exercise, meditation, or deep breathing exercises; healthy food choices; limited alcohol intake; a positive attitude; supportive friends; stress-management; and avoidance of unnecessary household and environmental chemicals.

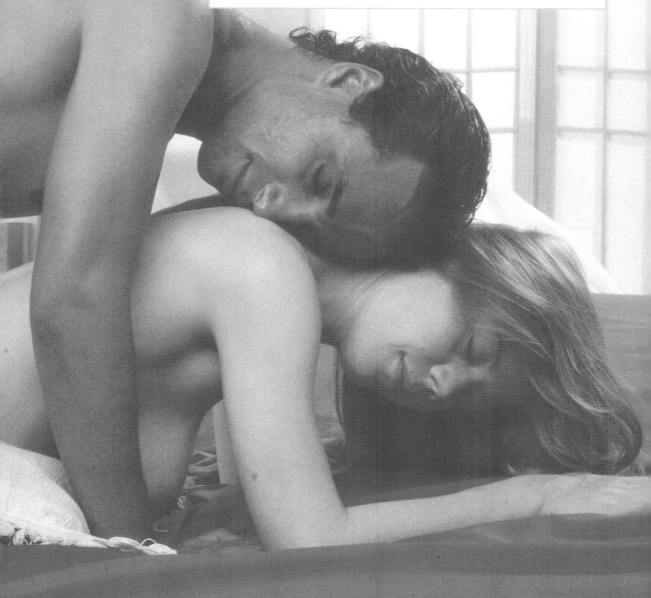

BENEFIT THE BODY • DAO TI

微 體

CONDITION According to the Chinese, when a woman's chi doesn't adequately reach and nourish the genitals, a woman can experience itching, discharge, or an unpleasant odor. Dao Ti massages the vagina and vaginal canal, which stimulates the flow of chi and improves vaginal function.

CURE HOW-TO The woman lies on her back, bending her legs at the knees and raising them toward her chest. The man holds his weight with his hands and feet. He inserts his penis, then withdraws it fully, performing this movement a total of 72 times.

FREQUENCY Eight times a day for 10 days.

FOCUS BOX

According to Chinese thought, the backbone is the path chi travels to reach the brain, from where it spreads to the rest of the body. Because Dao Ti creates a straight line from the man's penis to a woman's backbone, chi is transferred more powerfully in this position than in any other. To ensure optimum effectiveness, the woman's back should remain straight. A straight back is also essential in other chi-building pursuits, such as qi gong and tai chi; a bent or curved back will cause it to take longer for the chi to flow through the body.

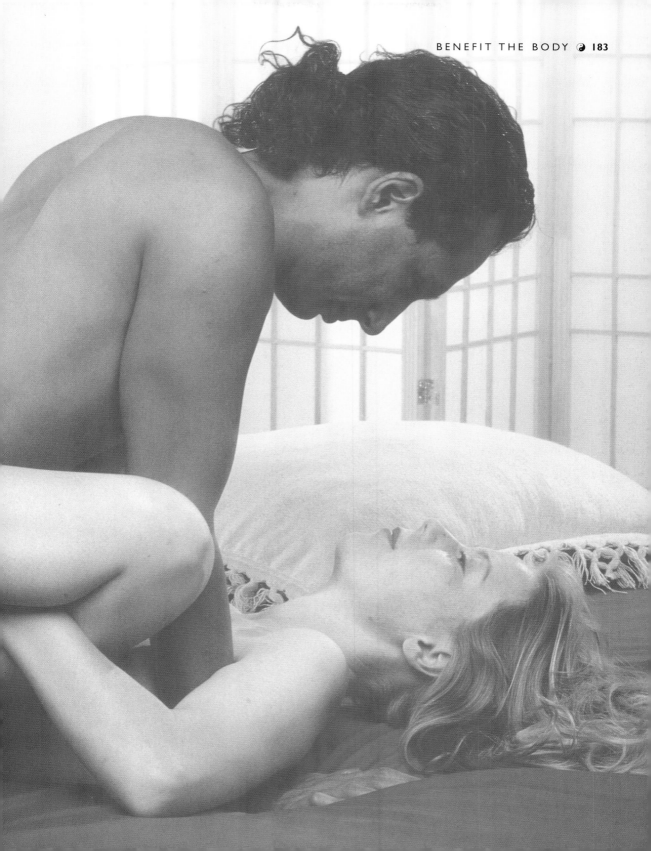

GLOSSARY

BALANCE Also called harmony. In Chinese medicine, good health results from the balance and harmonious interaction of yin and yang energies.

BUDDHISM Though it played an important role in ancient China, Buddhism was actually founded in Northern India in the sixth century B.C. by Siddhartha Gautama, who became known as the Buddha (Enlightened One). The Buddha achieved enlightenment (Nirvana) through meditation and established a community of monks to follow his example and encourage others. Buddhism teaches that Nirvana can be reached through meditation and good moral and religious behavior. Buddhist belief is centered around Four Noble Truths: all living beings must suffer; desire and self-importance cause suffering; the achievement of Nirvana ends suffering; and Nirvana can be attained through meditation and righteous actions, thoughts, and attitudes. While there are many different types of Buddhism, Zen Buddhism is the most prevalent in China. The name 'Zen' is derived from the Chinese Chan'an-na, which is a corruption of the Buddhist Dhyana, meaning 'meditation.'

CHANNELS Also called meridians. Channels are the nonmaterial pathways that run through the body and are connected to specific organs. Chi travels through channels.

CHI Pronounced 'chee' and alternately called 'qi,' 'energy,' 'vital energy,' 'primal energy,' and 'the life force,' chi is the fundamental energy found in all living things. For good health, peace of mind, and even conception, this energy must circulate unimpeded throughout the body.

CONFUCIANISM Founded by Chiu Kong (c. 551-479 B.C.), who was also called Kong the Philosopher, or K'ung Fu-tse. Confucius, as he is known today, emphasized the importance of 'li' (proper behavior), 'jen' (sympathetic attitude), and 'xiao' (ancestor worship).

ENERGY See 'Chi.'

FIVE ELEMENTS SYSTEM Also called the Five Phases. A system that organizes all processes in nature into five categories: Wind, Fire, Earth, Metal, and Water. Illness is also classified according to these five categories.

HARMONY See 'Balance.'

IMBALANCE A term commonly used in Chinese medicine to characterize illness, which the Chinese believe results from an imbalance of yin and yang energies or an imbalance of chi within the body.

JADE PRAYER MAT Also called *Carnal Prayer Mat*, this fictional morality tale was written during the Ming dynasty (A.D. 1368-1644), and admonishes readers against the dangers of wanton sex.

JIN PING MEI A book of fictional poetry celebrating sex, *Jin Ping Mei* was written during the Ming dynasty (A.D. 1368-1644). The poems tell the story of a wealthy man who married three women: Jin, Ping, and Mei.

LADY SU Among the earliest-known Taoist proponents of sex-for-health was a woman named Su Nu, also known as the Elemental Maid or Lady Su. Su Nu wrote a book during the first century A.D. that became known alternatively as *The Book of Lady Su* and *The Classic of the Elemental Lady*.

MERIDIAN See 'Channels.'

ORGANS In Chinese medicine, organs embody complex energy systems that are crucial to many functions within the body.

ORGAN CHI The chi energy unique to each organ and organ function. In illness, an organ's chi may be deficient, stagnant, overabundant, or hyperactive, depending on the specific yin or yang imbalance.

PENG ZU CHING Written during the rule of the Yellow

Emperor, c. 2700 B.C.,
Peng Zu Ching was based on the true story of Peng Zu, a man who appeared 50 years old when he was 100.

SURFACE CHI Also called 'Protective Chi.' The chi that circulates on the outside of the body to protect it from illnesses and imbalances caused by external or climatic conditions.

TAOISM Attributed to a philosopher named Laozi (also known as Li Erh or Lao Tzu) who lived during the Chou dynasty (c. 580 B.C.). An officer of the royal library, Laozi was said to roam the earth in the presence of a dragon. After years of study he became enlightened and decided to retreat from society, traveling to far-Western China on a water buffalo. Upon reaching a distant mountain pass, Laozi met the Keeper of the Pass, Wen-Shih, who convinced Laozi to record his insights in what became known as the *Tao Te Ching* (also called the *Dao De Jing*). Also called the Tao or Dao (which means 'the way'), the book of philosophy is a kind of manual of meditation and self-transformation.

YANG One of the two fundamental polar energies found in all living things. Yang qualities include hotness, dryness, and excess. Yang means 'the sun,' or 'the light side of a mountain.'

YELLOW EMPEROR
Huang Ti, who ascended to the throne in 2697 B.C.. Known later as the Yellow Emporer, Huang Ti was reported to be so interested in strengthening and maintaining his health—reportedly to please the estimated 1200 women whom he slept with during his lifetime— that he commissioned a team of six doctors to work with him on a book of medicine called *The Yellow Emperor's Classic of Internal Medicine*.

YELLOW EMPEROR INNER JING Also called *Huant Ti Nei Chin*, *Nei Ching*, and *The Yellow Emperor's Classic of Internal Medicine* this book was written by the Yellow Emperor Huang Ti and a team of doctors. It is considered the first book of Chinese medicine. In it are theories of yin and yang, the five elements, chi and chi meridians, and acupressure and acupuncture.

YIN One of the two fundamental polar energies found in all living things. Yin qualities include coldness, dampness, and deficiency. In addition to 'the moon,' yin alternatively means 'the dark side of a mountain.'

YIN AND YANG A Chinese theory of two mutually interdependent and constantly interacting opposite energies that sustain all living organisms. The interaction of yin and yang produces chi. Yin and yang is a particularly Chinese concept, one that denotes the two opposing forces that exist within every living thing. While yin and yang is often explained simply as contrary energies, the principle is actually more complex: Everything contains and is balanced by its own mutually dependent, polar opposite. The concept is symbolized by the sun and the moon—the two opposing forces active in our world—and is often depicted as a two-toned circle. Within the dark half of the circle lies a small light dot, and within the light half lies a small dark dot. This suggests that, though opposites, there is a necessary relationship between yin and yang. Neither exists in and of itself.

YIN AND YANG METHOD The Chinese term for health-supportive sex. The yin and yang method has been used in China since before the appearance of written language. The concept first appeared in print, however, late in the Zhou dynasty (c. 1027-256 B.C.), when philosophers refined the concept of yin and yang and created the related theory of duality, encompassing heaven and earth, sun and moon, man and woman.

MORE INFORMATION

BOOKS

Molony, David and Ming Ming Pan Molony. *American Association of Oriental Medicine's Complete Guide to Chinese Herbal Medicine: How to Treat Illness and Maintain Wellness with Chinese Herbs.* New York: Berkeley Publishing Group, 1998.

Wong, Eva. *Harmonizing Yin and Yang: The Dragon–Tiger Classic.* Boston: Shambhala Publications, 1997.

ORGANIZATIONS

AMERICAN FOUNDATION OF TRADITIONAL CHINESE MEDICINE
505 Beach Street
San Francisco, CA 94133
(415) 776-0502

JOURNAL OF CHINESE MEDICINE
c/o Eastland Press
1260 Activity Drive, #A
Vista, CA 92083
(800) 453-3278

JOURNAL OF ORIENTAL MEDICINE IN AMERICA
16161 Ventura Boulevard, Suite 406
Encino, CA 91436
(888) 556-5662

ORIENTAL HEALING ARTS INSTITUTE
1945 Palo Verde Avenue, Suite 208
Long Beach, CA 90815

THE HEALING TAO CENTER
P.O. Box 1194
Huntington, NY 11743
(516) 367-2701

TAOIST TAI CHI SOCIETY OF USA
1060 Bannock Street
Denver, CO 80204
(303) 623-5163

QI GONG INSTITUTE EAST-WEST ACADEMY OF THE HEALING ARTS
450 Sutter Street, Suite 916
San Francisco, CA 94108
(415) 788-2227

WEBSITES

YAK RIDER HYPERLINK
www.yakrider.com

ZAIHONG SHEN'S FENG SHUI NEW YORK
www.fengshuinewyork.com

GREAT TAO FOUNDATION OF AMERICA
www.taoism.net

HELPING PEOPLE SURVIVE ONLINE
www.hps-online.com/hsex.htm

ORIENTAL MEDICINE
www.orientalmedicine.com

TAO MANOR
www.home.earthlink.net/~gr8dao/

TAOIST RESTORATION SOCIETY
www.taorestore.org

INDEX

ACKNOWLEDGMENTS

PICTURE CREDITS

The publishers would like to thank the following for their kind permission to reproduce the photographs:

P21 The Ancient Art and Architecture Collection
P26-27 Christie's Images/Private Collection/The Bridgeman Art Library
P32 center left: Michael Yamashita/Colorific
P32 center: Brian Cosgrove
P32 center right: Tom Nebbia/Corbis
P32 B Ashe/Trip
P34 Chris Bradley/Axiom Photographic Agency
P35 top center: John Chard/gettyone stone
P35 top right: The Purcell Team/Corbis
P35 center: Ernst Haas/gettyone stone
P35 below left: Eddie Soloway/gettyone stone
P35 bottom center: Robert Harding Picture Library
P35 bottom right: Nasa
P37 top right: Lowell Georgia/Corbis
P37 bottom left: Chris Bradley/Axiom Photographic Agency
P37 bottom right: Brian Vikander/Corbis
P39 Lewis Kemper/gettyone stone
P52 Jake Fitzjones/Houses and Interiors
P53 Angela Wyant/gettyone stone
P154 Phil Schermeister/Corbis

Thanks to Dorling Kindersley photographers:
Peter Cadwick, Brian Cosgrove, Andy Crawford, Antonia Deutsch, Philip Dowell, Steve Gorto, Danuta Mayer, Max Alexander, Stephen Oliver, Andrew McKinney, Steven Wooster

AUTHOR'S ACKNOWLEDGMENTS

Even after five-thousand years of civilization, sex is still considered taboo in China. Having open-minded parents helped me see things far differently from the Confucian society which I grew up in. Thanks to my mother and father, I have been able to appreciate the role of sex in my own health and relationships.

I would like to thank my friends who have helped me write this book. J. Jurado, Stan Nadel, and Mari Allan, your editing was an invaluable step forward for me, and to Kenny Hui who encouraged me for publishing. To Chris Allan, who is a very special person in my life, and whose insight has helped me to cope with and grow through the difficult "culture-shock" which I have encountered while living in the West.

To my publishers at DK, LaVonne Carlson and Sean Moore, I am especially lucky to have benefited from your attention to elegant design and your commitment to bringing a highly regarded science of the East to the people of the West. To Stephanie Pederson, for her talent of transfering these ancient eastern beliefs to the western audience. To Barbara Berger for her great effort of coordinating the whole project. To Dirk Kaufman, for a brilliant cover design and for engaging with me in this project right from the start. To Tina Vaughan, who has the artistic vision of a beautiful package. To Claire Legamah, whose design style is absolutely elegant, from the structure layout to color selection. To Kellie Walsh, a photographer who has the eye to catch the perfect picture. To Mandy Earey who worked with patience and diligence to set up the photo studio and work with the models. To the make up and hair designer Tomami Mihara who was very patient during the endless shoot hours. And to all the models, for their professional devotion to the project.